Dukan Diet Cookbook

Over 100 Proven, Easy & Delicious Dukan Diet Recipes.
21 Day Four Phase Plan Included.

MICHAEL SMITH

Special Bonus

Ready to receive over 600 Delicious & Easy Recipes for FREE?

We want to thank you for purchasing the book and we hope to make your belly happy with the recipes that follow. As a token of our appreciation we have a little gift for you.

We are a team of small but passionate cookbook writers and our mission is to make cooking fun, simple and delicious. Writing recipes gives us a chance to have fun, be creative and let other people know that healthy and delicious food does not have to be complicated nor take hours and hours.

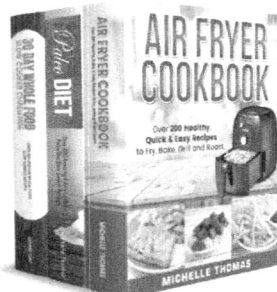

Only sign up for the cookbook box set if you are ready to be absolutely amazed with over 600 proven, delicious and easy to make recipes.

To access the gift page type in www.bit.ly/2Ho82AH or email us at info@limitlessrecipes.com to get the box set delivered to your email.

Limitless Recipes
Like us on Facebook and join our private Facebook group community for more recipes and gifts.

@limitlessrecipes
Follow us on Instagram

Limitless Recipes
Follow us on Pinterest.

Want to be a part of our closed Facebook group?
We are working on building an engaged community discussing recipes and healthy eating in our closed Facebook group. If you would like to be involved in the discussions about cooking, what is working, what is not working and receive information about gifts and promotions, we would be delighted to add you.

Type in Limitless Recipes on Facebook or write us at info@limitlessrecipes.com. Come say hi!

Happy Cooking!

Table of Contents

Introduction

The Dukan Diet is a high-protein, low-fat eating regimen devised in 2010 by Pierre Dukan, a French nutritionist. It is an eating habit that aims to help a person lose excess weight by reducing carbohydrate consumption in a natural manner, thus reducing calorie intake.

The method helps boosts a body's metabolism rate. It also normalizes and balances the energy consumption and usage, which the Dukan Diet claims cause obesity and overweight. The eating regimen consists of the following 4 phases.

Before you start your journey to your Dukan Diet, I recommend that you first get a food journal to keep track of your food intake and progress. Get BookFactory Food Journal (Link to Amazon: https://amzn.to/2YilHyH).

Phase I: The Attack – Pure Protein (PP)

The first phase of the diet involves consuming protein and nothing else and aims to trigger ketogenesis, a process wherein you teach the body to use fat instead of glucose (simple sugar) and utilizes the by-product, ketones, a source of energy.

This phase can last from 2 up to 7 days, depending on how much weight you have to lose. The guidelines are as follows:

* 1 up to 2 days for 10 pounds
* 3 up to 5 days for 30 pounds
* 7 up to 10 days for more than 40 pounds, and only with the advice of your physician

During this stage, you are allowed to consume an unlimited amount approved 68 types of animal protein, which some studies proved to produce a satiating effect and help speed up weight reduction.

Physical Activity

Being active will optimize your weight loss goals. You can take a 25-minute of walk every day in the morning to maintain a healthy physical activity – it has many benefits, costs nothing, and natural.

Daily Oat Bran Intake

Taking a sufficient amount of oat-bran every day is vital in the Dukan Diet. It provides your body with some carbohydrates and needed fiber to bind the food calories you eat and help limit absorption. During this phase, you have to take 1 1/2 tablespoons every day.

Daily Fluid Intake

During this phase, the ketogenic process will flush out excess amounts of water from the body, so it is vital that you drink 6 up to 8 cups or at least 1 1/2 liters of water every day. You can use it in your coffee, herbal tea, or plain tea.

Phase II: The Cruise – Proteins & Vegetables (PV)

After you jump-started and sped up your metabolism and weight loss, this stage reintroduces 32 kinds of non-starchy, low-carbohydrate vegetables to include in your food base that you can consume, along with the 68 approved proteins.

You must follow a very exact timescale during this stage, which is 3 days for every 1 pound of weight you lose. For example, if you lost 20 pounds, you must follow the guidelines for 60 days, or till you achieve your True Weight.

The 100 kinds of approved foods that you can eat in unlimited amounts in this phase will help you maintain steady, but gradual weight loss, around an average of 1 pound every 3 days, until you reach your True Weight. Due to their diversity, they will also supply your body with fiber, minerals, and vitamins.

Alternating Menu Rhythm
During this stage, you will have to choose alternating PV and PP rhythm that suits your lifestyle. You can choose to have 1 day of PP followed by 1 day of PP or 1:1 ratio. If you have lots of excess weight to lose or if you are not losing any weight you can choose 2 day2 of PP followed by 2 day2 of PP, and even increase the ratio to 3:3, 4:4, or 5:5. The 5 days PP and 5 days PV is especially recommended for a person who has too much excess weight to lose.

Physical Activity
Take a 30-minute of brisk walk every day to maintain a healthy physical activity.

Daily Oat Bran Intake
* 2 tablespoons every day

Tolerated Food
During this phase, you are allowed to use the following items. Take note of their indicated serving size.

* 3 drops olive oil
* 2 tablespoons of wine (white or red)
* 1 tablespoon cornstarch daily, or use agar-agar as a thickener (1 tbsp. for every 1 cup water, or according to the recipe needs
* 1 tablespoon soy sauce daily
* 1 tablespoon cocoa powder (non-fat, unsweetened) daily
* meat cube (non-fat)

* 1 tablespoon ketchup (unsweetened) daily
* Maximum of 30 grams of cheeses (6% fat)
* 1 tablespoon cream (non-fat)
* Maximum of 150 grams rhubarb daily
You may also use Protein Rich Food Supplement to boost effects on your body. You may buy Muscle Milk (Link to Amazon: https://amzn.to/2YeGK5c) and Quest Protein Powder (Link to Amazon: https://amzn.to/2YiyNvV)

Phase III: The Consolidation

After you reached your True Weight, this phase will help you avoid gaining back the weight you lost. You must follow a very exact timescale during this stage, which is 5 days for every 1 pound of weight you lose. For example, if you lost 20 pounds, you must follow the guidelines for 100 days.

During this period you need to eat the 100 kinds of approved foods. Basically, you have PV as your food base every day. Plus, you can reintroduce approved foods in your menu following a strict guideline.

For example, for the total of 100 days, if you lost 20 pounds, you can eat allowed servings of approved foods every day or week for 50 days, and consume allowed servings for the rest of the phase. You can add the following to your menu:

First half of the phase additions	Second half of the phase additions
1 serving approved fruit daily	2 servings approved fruit daily
2 slices bread (whole-grain) daily	2 slices bread (whole-grain) daily
1 1/2 ounces cheese (hard rind)	1 1/2 ounces cheese (hard rind)
1 cooked cup-serving starchy food weekly	2 cooked cups-serving starchy food weekly
1 celebration meal weekly	1 celebration meal weekly

For the celebration meal, you can consume 1 glass of your favorite wine, 1 dessert, 1 entrée, and 1 appetizer.

Pure Protein Thursday
Together with the guideline mentioned above, you also need to have a PP day every Thursday to help you maintain your True Weight and avoid gaining back the weight you lost.

Physical Activity
Take a 25-minute of brisk walk every day to maintain a healthy physical activity.

Daily Oat Bran Intake
* 2 tablespoons every day

Phase IV: The Stabilization

The final stage of the diet aims to stabilize your True Weight for the remainder of your life. In theory, you are allowed to eat whatever food you want after you succeed in the first 3 phases. However, you must continue to practice your new eating habit so you do not regain the weight you lose.

During this phase, you must do the following the following simple rules. They are non-negotiable to help you retain your successful weight loss.

* Consume 3 tablespoons of oat bran daily.
* Be physically active whenever you can, like taking the stairs.
* Keep the PP day every Thursday.

Top 5 Secrets to Get Slim with Ease

In a fast-paced world, it is not always easy to follow an eating habit with guidelines and rules, especially when on a diet. Here are some tips that can help you lose weight while following the Dukan Diet.

I. Season Your Dishes

Condiments, herbs, and spices add not just new dimensions into your dishes, but flavorful recipes also make even the simplest meals wonderful, especially during the PP phase. You can mix ginger with shrimp, cinnamon with chicken, vanilla with white fish, and more. Explore cuisines from other countries. They may provide you wonderful recipes that use the ingredients that are on the 100 approved foods.

II. Take Advantage of the Variety and Seasonal Foods

Adopt your menu to include the available lean proteins on PP days, vegetables on PV days, and fruits and starchy veggies on the Consolidation Phase that are available to buy for the season.

You will receive the maximum nutritional benefits by eating a wide variety of foods that are included in the list of 100 approved types for the diet. Frozen, plain veggies will take less time to prepare and to cook. Moreover, find creative ways to incorporate oat bran on your daily menu. You can do any of the following to consume your needed intake:

- make oat bran porridge with milk
- stir 1 up to 2tablespoons in your stews of soups
- mix 1 up to 2tablespoons in your cottage cheese, yogurt, or omelets,
- use an equal amount of it as breading for cooking instead of breadcrumbs
- use as a topping for casserole instead of breadcrumbs
- breading for fish and chicken, or
- sprinkle 1 up to 2 tablespoons on your salads

Moreover, you can also incorporate wheat bran into your baked goods and meals. Here are a few ways you can use or add it to your diet:

- add 2 tablespoons up to 1/2 cup of it in various bread, pancake, waffle, dinner roll, and muffin recipes
- sprinkle on cold or hot cereals
- stir 1 up to 2 tablespoons in your stews and soups, or
- mix it with your breading mix to coat veggies, fish, or meat for baking or sautéing

III. Use Tolerated Items Wisely
During the PV phase, as well as the Stabilization phase, where you are allowed to consume 2 tolerated items daily, choose which ones to use because of their fat and carbohydrate content.

IV: Techniques to Cook Dishes without Fats
You will use limited to no fat when you are on the Dukan Diet, but there are methods to help you cook them well. Marinate your protein in various spices herbs, salt, soy sauce, lemon, etc. before grilling to tenderize them.

Use silicone molds (Link to Amazon: https://amzn.to/2HBoQV7) for baking cakes and muffins, nonstick pots and pans (Link to Amazon: https://amzn.to/2JBcH4z), line cooking containers with parchment papers for pies, cookies, and tarts, and bake using foil dishes (Link to Amazon: https://amzn.to/2CDtiP7). Microwave or steam your meals.

V. White Day
If you are experiencing problems in losing weight or if your weight loss has stopped, do a "White Day" to help you pass the hurdle. Consume white fish, white meat or chicken, white egg, and yogurt.

BONUS TIP: Substitute Ingredients
You can check your favorite dishes and see if you can substitute any of the ingredients with approved ones. You may be able to enjoy them as dishes in your diet if you can do any or all of the following:

* Oat bran, powdered milk (fat-free), Konjac powder, Agar-agar, or cornstarch for flour
* Shirataki noodles for pastas
* Seasonal vegetables for potatoes
* Low fat for regular cheese
* Skim milk for cream
* Use fat-free cheese or silken tofu
* Greek yogurt (plain, fat-free) for cream and butter
* Herbs and spices, such as shallots, peppercorns, dill, etc.

** If you cannot find quark cheese in your area, then you can substitute with yogurt (plain, fat-free) with preferred herbs or fromage frais.

21 Day Action Plan

Here is a simple menu that you can follow to kick-start your Dukan Diet.

Attack Phase: Pure Protein

Do not forget your intake of 1 1/2 tablespoons oat bran and drink 6 up to 8 cups of water every day, as well as your daily exercise.

Snack options:
- A couple slices turkey
- 1 serving yogurt (fruit-flavored, fat-free)
- Eggs (hard-boiled)
- Cold chicken slices
- Jelly (sugar-jelly)
- Any appetizer dishes can be served as snack, if desired
- Leftovers of recipes, if any

WEEK I

Day 1:
Breakfast: Oat Bran Muffins 21
Lunch: Beef Rosemary Burgers p. 34
Dinner: Chicken Kebabs p. 36

Day 2:
Breakfast: Yogurt 31
Lunch: Salmon Pancakes p. 25
Dinner: Fishcake p. 34

Day 3:
Breakfast: Milk & Muesli p. 24
Lunch: Ham Balls p. 27
Dinner: Herbed Baked Fish 33

Day 4:
Breakfast: Smoked Salmon Scrambled Eggs 25
Lunch: Oat Bran Pancake 32
Dinner: Mustard Dill Sauced Salmon Escalopes 35

Day 5:
Breakfast: Oat Bran Porridge 19
Lunch: Egg & Prawn Salad 23
Dinner: Vietnamese Beef 29

Cruise Phase: Alternating Pure Protein & Protein Vegetables (1:1)

Do not forget your intake of 1 1/2 tablespoons of oat bran every day, as well as your daily exercise.

Snack options:
- A couple slices turkey
- 1 serving yogurt (fruit-flavored, fat-free), sprinkled with oat bran if desired
- Eggs (hard-boiled)
- Cold chicken slices
- Jelly (sugar-jelly)
- Carrot sticks
- String cheese (mozzarella, non-fat)
- Cheddar (non-fat)
- Philly cheese (non-fat)
- Any appetizer dishes can be served as snack, if desired
- Leftovers of recipes, if any

Day 6: PP
Breakfast: High-Protein Vanilla & Rum-Flavored Pancakes   24
Lunch: Chicken or Turkey Zen Balls   22
Dinner: Garlicky Prime Rib   26

Day 7: PV
Breakfast: Leek & Smoked Salmon Scramble   62
Lunch: Turkey Meatballs   23
Dinner: Salmon & Herbed Oat Bran-Broccoli Tabbouleh   40

WEEK II
Day 8: PP
Breakfast: Blueberry Muffins   25
Lunch: Peppery Halibut Steaks   26
Dinner: Seared Tuna & Arugula   55

Day 9: PV
Breakfast: Cheesy Spinach Muffins   55
Lunch: Easy Stir-Fry Seafood   43
Dinner: Barbequed Cod & Wilted Spinach   41

Day 10: PP
Breakfast: Oat Bran-Egg White Galette   29
Lunch: Fast Garlic Shrimp   30
Dinner: Yogurt & Aleppo Pepper-Marinated Chicken Kebabs   27

Day 11: PV
Breakfast: Pumpkin Muffins 57
Lunch: Easy Stir-Fry Seafood 43
Dinner: Red Wine Stewed Beef 60

Day 12: PP
Breakfast: Cheesy Omelet 30
Lunch: Lemony Chicken Cutlets 31
Dinner: Baby Back Ribs 28

Day 13: PV
Breakfast: Bacon Scrambled Egg 58
Lunch: Mustard Chicken & Baked Tomatoes 39
Dinner: Smoked Salmon & Cabbage Salad 42

Day 14: PP
Breakfast: Herbed Omelet 32
Lunch: Peppery Halibut Steaks 26
Dinner: Garlicky Prime Rib 26

WEEK III
Day 15: PV
Breakfast: Leek & Smoked Salmon Scramble 62
Lunch: Shrimp-Stuffed Peppers 45
Dinner: Baked Monkfish and Tomato Loaf 44

Day 16: PP
Breakfast: Oat Bran Muffins
Lunch: Beef Rosemary Burgers
Dinner: Chicken Kebabs

Day 17: PV
Breakfast: Cheesy Spinach Muffins 21
Lunch: Baked Provencal Cod 45
Dinner: Seafood Skewers & Vegetable Medley 53

Day 18: PP
Breakfast: Yogurt 31
Lunch: Salmon Pancakes 25
Dinner: Fishcake 34

Day 19: PV
Breakfast: Pumpkin Muffins 57
Lunch: Shrimp Green Chili 54
Dinner: Herbed Cod Packets 51

Day 20: PP
Breakfast: Milk & Muesli 24
Lunch: Ham Balls 27
Dinner: Herbed Baked Fish 33

Day 21: PV
Breakfast: Leek & Smoked Salmon Scramble 62
Lunch: Seared Tuna & Arugula 55
Dinner: Vegetable & Marinated Beef Kebabs 54

If you really are serious about Dukan Diet, I recommend that you buy the bestseller book for Dukan Diet: The Dukan Diet Paperback (Link to Amazon paperback: https://amzn.to/2HJjLdD and link to Amazon audiobook: https://amzn.to/2HInoQS. The free audiobook applies only if you don't have an audible account. You can get two books for free and the books are yours to keep even if you cancel the free trial.

My favourite tools for cooking are the following items: Philips Airfryer, with Fat Removal Technology Black (Link to Amazon: https://amzn.to/2YpuCyk) and Instant Pot Pressure Cooker (Link to Amazon: https://amzn.to/2FC0zeq)

You can also take Dukan Diet capsules to supplement your diet program. Dukan Diet Appetite and Fat Control (Link to Amazon: https://amzn.to/2V0gUA2). Always consult your doctor before taking any prescriptions.

ATTACK PHASE (PP)

Poultry Muffins

Appetizer: Servings|6   Prep. Time|**20 minutes**   Cook Time|**15 minutes**
Nut. Content (per serving): Cal|**243**   Fat|**8.3g**   Protein|**37.3g**   Carbs|**3.7g**

1 cup chicken or turkey breast, chopped finely in your food processor
1 teaspoon baking powder
1 teaspoon mustard (Dijon)
1/4 cup creamy cheese (pre-mixed)
2 tablespoons herbs (fresh), chopped, optional

2 tablespoons pickled peppers (pre-mixed), optional
2 teaspoons hot sauce (Sriracha), optional
3 eggs (medium), separated
3 tablespoon oat bran, preferably oat bran (organic, Dukan Diet)

1. Preheat your oven to 350F. Grease a 12-cup, nonstick muffin pan with 1/8 teaspoon olive oil, or line them with baking cups (parchment paper).
2. Separate the eggs, placing the yolks and whites in different mixing bowls. Whisk the whites till stiff peaks form. Add the rest of the ingredients to the bowl with the yolks; stir to mix well. Carefully fold the white and yolk mixture till mixed.
3. With a soup spoon, scoop the batter into the prepared muffin cups; filling each section around 3/4 full. Bake in the oven for 15 minutes. When done, transfer to a cooling rack; let sit for 5 to Ten (10) minutes before removing the muffins from the mold. Transfer the muffins to a cooling rack; let them cool.

Oat Bran Porridge   p.15

Breakfast: Servings|1   Prep. Time|**5 to Ten (10) minutes**   Cook Time|**2 minutes**
Nut. Content (per serving): Cal|**123**   Fat|**1.4g**   Protein|**11g**   Carbs|**22.1g**

2 tablespoons oat bran
A bit of wheat bran

1 cup milk (skim), adjust to preference
Sweetener, adjust to preference

1. Mix all of the ingredients; microwave for 2 minutes.

Herbed Chicken Omelet Sandwich

Main Dish: Servings|**1**   Prep. Time|**5 minutes**   Cook Time|**4 minutes**
Nut. Content (per serving): Cal|**722**   Fat|**43.8g**   Protein|**65.7g**   Carbs|**18.6g**

1 chicken breast, cooked & shredded
1 tab espoon cream cheese (fat-free)
1 tablespoon parsley, chopped
1 teaspoon baking powder

2 tablespoons yogurt (Greek, plain, fat-free)
3 eggs
3 tablespoons oat bran

1. In a microwavable bowl (rectangular), mix the egg, yogurt, baking powder, and oat bran till even y combined. Sprinkle the parsley on top; microwave on HIGH for 4 minutes. Remove from the microwave; let cool till set like bread. Cut into 2 bread-like slices; very tightly toast to prevent them from over-drying.
2. Whisk the eggs with your preferred herbs (chopped). Grease a frying pan (nonstick) with a couple drops of olive oil. Add the egg mixture; fry like an omelet. When cooked, fold the 4 sides in to create a rectangle.
3. Evenly spread the cream cheese on each slice of oat bran bread. Put a chicken on one slice, top with the omelet, and then cover with the second slice. Serve.

Tahitian Flan

Dessert: Servings|**1**   Prep. Time|**5 minutes**   Cook Time|**4 minutes**
Nut. Content (per serving): Cal|**189**   Fat|**9.9g**   Protein|**13.2g**   Carbs|**11.5g**

1 egg
1 teaspoon coconut extract
1/2 cup evaporated milk (fat-free)

1 teaspoon Splenda or stevia (granulated sweetener), adjust to preference, preferably organic stevia (Dukan Diet)

1. Directly in a microwavable bowl (single-serving) or ramekin, break the eggs. Add the coconut extract and sweetener; briefly whisk to mix. Add the milk over the mixture.
2. Place the container on a microwavable plate; microwave for 4 minutes on MEDIUM power. Remove from the oven. Immediately transfer to a rimmed baking tray filled with water (ice cold) to cool the flan quickly. Serve.

Creamed Coffee Custard

Dessert: Servings|2   Prep. Time|**5 minutes**   Cook Time **Ten (10) minutes**
Nut. Content (per serving): Cal|**231**   Fat|**9.9g**   Protein|**13.5g**   Carbs|**22.2g**

1 cup milk (fat-free)
2 eggs
2 tablespoons coffee granules (instant)

2 tablespoons Splenda or stevia (granulated sweetener), adjust to preference, preferably organic stevia (Dukan Diet)

1. In a saucepan (small), add the coffee and milk; let come to boil and then remove from the heat. In a bowl (clean), beat the eggs using a whisk. Add about 2 tablespoons milk into the beaten eggs; stir to temper. While constantly stirring, add the rest of the milk mixture.
2. Transfer the egg mixture to the same saucepan. While constantly stirring, heat for Ten (10) minutes or till thick, letting it come to a boil in the process. Once the mixture coated the back of a wooden spoon, remove the pan from heat. Sweeten to preference. Divide between serving dishes. Refrigerate for at least 2 hours or till chilled. Serve.

Coffee Granita

Dessert: Servings|4   Prep. Time **Ten (10) minutes**   Cook Time|**5 minutes**
Nut. Content (per serving): Cal|**44**   Fat|**0.1g**   Protein|**0.3g**   Carbs|**11g**

1 cup espresso (prepared) or coffee (very strong)
2 cups water
2 tablespoons milk (fat-free)

3 tablespoons Splenda or stevia (granulated sweetener), adjust to preference, preferably organic stevia (Dukan Diet)

1. In a saucepan, heat the milk, water, and sweetener on low heat till the sweetener is fully dissolve; let come to a boil. Once boiling, remove from the heat; let cool. Once cool, stir in the coffee/espresso; transfer to a freezable container. Freeze for 1 hour.
2. To serve, briefly run water on the outside of the container to loosen the granita. Transfer to a blender, pulse till the texture is crystal-like. Divide between 4 serving dishes. Serve right away.

Oat Bran Muffins

Dessert: Servings|4   Prep. Time|**10-15 minutes**   Cook Time|**20 to 30 minutes**
Nut. Content (per serving): Cal|**173**   Fat|**11g**   Protein|**12.5g**   Carbs|**11g**

1/2 teaspoon sweetener
4 eggs, separated
4 tablespoons fromage frais

8 tablespoons oat bran
Cinnamon or lemon zest

1. Preheat your oven to 180C. Whisk the egg whites till stiff peaks appear. Mix the rest of the ingredients till well blended. Fold the mixture into the egg whites. Pour into muffin cups; bake for 20 to 30 minutes.

Chicken or Turkey Zen Balls

Main Dish: Servings|**3**   Prep. Time|**20 minutes**   Cook Time|**0 minutes**
Nut. Content (per serving): Cal|**194**   Fat|**4.5g**   Protein|**33.9g**   Carbs|**3.3g**

1 tablespoon (pre-mixed) pickled pepper
1 tablespoon cream cheese (fat-free or low-fat)
1 teaspoon hot sauce (Sriracha), optional

1/2 cup chicken or turkey breast, cooked meat & chopped in your food processor.1 tablespoon oat bran, preferably Oat bran (organic, Dukan Diet), place in a different container if using as a coating

1. Put the cream cheese and meat in your food processor; process till minced. Fold in the pickled pepper. Roll the mixture into small balls, making 6 pieces. Roll each ball in the oat bran till coated. Keep refrigerated till serving time. Serve cold.

Jewel Egg Soup

Appetizer: Servings|**1**   Prep. Time|**2 minutes**   Cook Time **Ten (10) minutes**
Nut. Content (per serving): Cal|**189**   Fat|**011.8g**   Protein|**16.3g**   Carbs|**5.8g**

1 1/2 cups chicken stock (low sodium)
1 egg

1 tablespoon scallions, chopped
Pinch salt

1. Whisk the egg very well. Transfer into a frying pan (small) greased with 1/8 teaspoon olive oil; cook without disturbing.
2. Meanwhile, heat the stock in a saucepan. Add the scallions. Once the eggs are cooked, transfer to a slicing board; fold into a package. Transfer the egg package to the bowl. Add your stock. Serve while very hot.

Yogurt Orange Cake

Dessert: Servings|**4**   Prep. Time|**15 minutes**   Cook Time|**45 minutes**
Nut. Content (per serving): Cal|**159**   Fat|**8.1g**   Protein|**9.9g**   Carbs|**11.4g**

1/2 teaspoon artificial sweetener
150 grams of natural yogurt (fat-free)
1teaspoon orange extract
2 teaspoon yeast

3 drops vegetable oil
3 eggs
4 tablespoon corn flour

1. Preheat your oven to 180C. Whisk the yeast, corn flour, orange extract, sweetener, and yogurt till well blended. Transfer to a greased and parchment paper-lined cake tin. Bake for 45 minutes or till cooked through.

Tea Sorbet

Dessert: Servings|**2**   Prep. Time|**20 minutes**   Cook Time|**0 minutes**
Nut. Content (per serving): Cal|**70**   Fat|**0g**   Protein|**4.4g**   Carbs|**13.5g**

2 tablespoons lemon juice (fresh)
3 tablespoons black tea (loose)

4 mint leaves (fresh)

1. In a bowl (medium), mix the tea with 1 1/4 cup boiling water. Cover the bowl; let stand for 3 minutes to infuse. Strain 4 tablespoons of the tea-infused water into a freezable, flat dish; freeze, stirring the mixture occasionally till ice crystals begin to form.
2. Strain the rest of the tea-infused water through your strainer; add the lemon juice and mix. Pour the mixture in your ice cream machine; churn for 15 minutes or till frozen.
3. To serve, fill serving glasses with the sorbet, top with the ice crystals, and garnish with mint leaves.

Turkey Meatballs *16*

Entrée/Appetizer: Servings|**16 meatballs**   Prep. Time|**30 minutes**   Cook Time|**20 minutes**
Nut. Content (per ball): Cal|**87**   Fat|**4.2g**   Protein|**10g**   Carbs|**3g**

1 1/2 pounds ground turkey (preferably organic)
1 onion (medium), grated
1 teaspoon oregano (dried)
1/2 cup cottage cheese (non-fat)

1/2 cup mint (fresh), minced
1/4 cup oat bran
2 cloves garlic, minced
2 egg whites, beaten
Salt & pepper, adjust to preference

1. In a bowl (medium), mix all of the ingredients, making sure not to over mix or your meatballs will become tough. By 1 tablespoon-full, scoop the mixture and form into balls. Put the meatballs in a sheet pan lined with parchment paper; broil till they are brown, turning once in the process.

Egg & Prawn Salad

Lunch: Servings|**2**   Prep. Time|**15-20 minutes**   Cook Time|**6 minutes**
Nut. Content (per serving): Cal|**436**   Fat|**22.2g**   Protein|**22.4g**   Carbs|**40g**

1 teaspoon olive oil
200 grams prawns, cooked & shelled
4 eggs

4 teaspoons vinegar (cider)
600 grams lettuce
A few tarragon sprigs

1. Mix the pepper and salt to preference, vinegar, and oil. In a bowl, mix in the prawns, tarragon, and lettuce in a bowl. Cook the eggs for 6 minutes in boiling water till soft-boiled. Carefully remove the shells; the yolks will be runny. Dress the lettuce mixture and while the eggs are still hot, top them on the lettuce.

High-Protein Vanilla & Rum-Flavored Pancakes 16

Breakfast: Servings|**10 pancakes**   Prep. Time **Ten (10) minutes**   Cook Time|**5minutes**
Nut. Content (per serving): Cal|**205**   Fat|**10.2g**   Protein|**13.1g**   Carbs|**16g**

1 teaspoon vanilla flavoring
1/2 liter milk (skimmed)
10 tablespoons powdered protein (Protifar)
100 grams corn flour (tolerated)
4 eggs

2 tablespoons powdered sweetener, adjust to preference
20 drops melted butter flavoring
200 grams silken tofu
30 drops white rum flavoring

1. In a bowl, mix the eggs, protein powder, corn flour, and tofu. Add the flavorings; stir to mix. Add the milk; mix till the mixture is a smooth batter.
2. Heat a pan (nonstick), ladle a scoop of batter in the pan; cook till the underside is brown. Flip; continue cooking till done.
NOTES: Do not eat more than 2 pancakes per day.

Matcha Green Tea Madeleines

Dessert: Servings|**12**   Prep. Time **Ten (10) minutes**   Cook Time|**30 minutes**
Nut. Content (per serving): Cal|**48**   Fat|**1.8g**   Protein|**2.4g**   Carbs|**6.5g**

1 tablespoon sweetener (Splenda)
1/2 teaspoon baking powder
2 eggs
4 tablespoons oat bran (Dukan Diet)
3 tablespoons quark or fromage frais (0% fat)

2 teaspoons tea powder (Matcha green), or 15 drops almond, lemon, or preferred flavoring
3 tablespoons cornstarch (tolerated)

1. Preheat your oven to 180C. Mix the quark or fromage frais in a bowl. Add the baking powder, cornstarch, and oat bran; mix well. Add the green tea and sweetener; mix well.
Pour the batter into silicone molds. Bake for 20 to 30 minutes, making sure not to overcook them. Once cooked, remove them from the oven. Let cool for 2 hours at room temperature.

Milk & Muesli 18

Breakfast: Servings|**2**   Prep. Time|**20 minutes**   Cook Time|**30 minutes**
Nut. Content (per serving): Cal|**132**   Fat|**6g**   Protein|**08g**   Carbs|**19g**

1 egg
1 tablespoon liquid sweetener

6 tablespoon oat bran
Almond essence

1. Preheat your oven to 160C. Mix all of the ingredients till well blended. Spread the mixture in a baking paper-lined tray; bake for 30 minutes. Once cooked, let cool and crumble; Store in airtight containers.

Blueberry muffins 16

Breakfast: Servings|6   Prep. Time **Ten (10) minutes**   Cook Time|**30 minutes**
Nut. Content (per serving): Cal|**140**   Fat|**7.3g**   Protein|**9g**   Carbs|**13.8g**

1 teaspoon baking powder
12 tablespoons oat bran
2 tablespoons granulated sweetener
(Splenda)
2 teaspoons blueberry or cranberry
flavoring

4 eggs
4 heaping tablespoons goji berries, optional
4 tablespoons fromage frais (plain, fat-free),
or quark (fat-free)

1. Preheat your oven to 180C. Separate your egg yolks from the whites in different deep containers. Using an electric beater, beat the whites till soft peaks appear. Add the blueberry flavoring, oat bran, fromage frais, sweetener, and yolks; mix well. Divide the batter into muffin cups lined with paper liners. Bake for 30 minutes.
2. Once cooked, remove from the oven; let cool and then refrigerate for 2 hours before serving. You can serve them for Cruise Phase. Keep refrigerated for a couple of days or store in airtight freezable bags and freeze for longer storage.
3. Optional goji berries: Put the berries in a bowl (small), add some water, and few drops of the blueberry flavoring; let soak for 30 minutes till they are juicy and plump. Fold these into your mixture before baking.

Smoked Salmon Scrambled Eggs p. 15

Breakfast: Servings|**1**   Prep. Time|**5 to Ten (10) minutes**   Cook Time|**1 minute, 30 seconds**
Nut. Content (per serving): Cal|**349**   Fat|**23.3g**   Protein|**30g**   Carbs|**3g**

2 eggs
Splash of milk (skim)

1/4 cup smoked salmon, as much as
preferred

1. Whisk the milk and the eggs in a microwavable bowl till well blended. Add the salmon, stir to mix well. Microwave for 1 minute on HIGH. Stir and microwave for 30 seconds more. Serve.

Salmon Pancakes p. 15, 17

Lunch: Servings|**2**   Prep. Time **Ten (10) minutes**   Cook Time|**0 minutes**
Nut. Content (per serving): Cal|**596**   Fat|**23g**   Protein|**79g**   Carbs|**17g**

1 small jar salmon roe
2 oat bran pancakes, see recipe
300 grams fromage frais (fat-free)

4 salmon slices smoked
60 grams quark (fat-free)

1. Mix the roe, quark, and fromage frais in a bowl; season with pepper and salt to preference. Divide the mixture between the pancakes. Top each with the salmon.

Garlicky Prime Rib 16, 17

Main Dish: Servings|**10**   Prep. Time **Ten (10) minutes**   Cook Time|**1 1/2 hours**
Nut. Content (per serving): Cal|**185**   Fat|**16.3g**   Protein|**7.5g**   Carbs|**2.3g**

2 teaspoons thyme
2 teaspoons salt
2 teaspoons pepper
2 tablespoons olive oil

10 pounds beef roast (prime rib)
10 cloves garlic, crushed, top sliced off, peeled, & very finely diced

1. Put the garlic in a bowl (small). Add the pepper, salt, thyme, and olive oil; blend well till mixed. Put the ribs on a roasting pan (large) with the fatty-side above. Rub the fatty side with the garlic mixture; let rest for up to 1 hour at room temperature.
2. Preheat your oven to 500F. Roast the ribs for 20 minutes. Reduce the temperature to 325F; roast for 60 to 70 minutes. The meat is done when the internal temperature reaches 135F for medium-rare. Once cooked to desired doneness, remove from the oven; let rest for Fifteen to Twenty min. to redistribute the juices.
NOTES: Cooking the ribs on your oven for 500F during the first 20 minutes could burn your meat. If your oven is too hot, then reduce the temperature to 460 for 20 minutes instead.

Peppery Halibut Steaks 16, 17

Main Dish: Servings|**4**   Prep. Time| **Fifteen to Twenty min.**   Cook Time|**8 minutes**
Nut. Content (per serving): Cal|**337**   Fat|**25.3g**   Protein|**24.6g**   Carbs|**1.4g**

1 1/2 teaspoon olive oil
1 tablespoon black pepper (ground)
1 tablespoon lemon juice

3/4 teaspoon salt (sea)
4 pieces (6-ounce each) halibut fillets
Cooking spray

1. Preheat your grill to medium heat. In a bowl (small), mix the olive oil, lemon juice, salt, and black pepper. Rub the fish fillets with the oil mixture evenly and coat well; let marinate for Ten (10) minutes.
2. Grease the grill with the cooking spray. Add the fish; cook for 4 minutes each side or till just cooked through. Serve.

ν Yogurt & Aleppo Pepper-Marinated Chicken Kebabs /6

Main Dish: Servings|4   Prep. Time|**40 to 50 minutes**   Cook Time|**10 to 12 minutes**
Nut. Content (per serving): Cal|**420**   Fat|**17.3g**   Protein|**57g**   Carbs|**7g**

1 1/2 teaspoons Aleppo pepper
1 cup yogurt (Greek, low-fat)
1 teaspoon black pepper (ground)
2 1/4 pounds chicken (boneless & skinless),
cubed into 1 1/4-inch chunk
2 lemons
2 tablespoons natural ketchup (sugar-free)

2 tablespoons vinegar (red wine)
3 tablespoons olive oil
3 teaspoons salt (kosher)
6 cloves garlic, crushed & peeled
Cooking spray or preferred oil for greasing
the grill

1. Put the pepper in a bowl (large) or your blender. Add 1 tablespoon lukewarm water; let sit for 5 minutes or till the texture is a thick paste. Add the garlic, yogurt, pepper, salt, ketchup, vinegar, and olive oil; mix well.
2. Slice the lemons into rounds or coins. Add to the marinade. Add the chicken; toss to coat well. Marinate in your fridge for a maximum of 24 hours. Once marinated, skewer the chicken chunks.
3. Brush the grill with a bit of oil and preheat to medium-high heat. Once heated, add the kebabs; cook for 10 to 12 minutes or till cooked through, turning them occasionally.
NOTES: If using a yogurt that is not thick, pour it on a thin cheesecloth-lined strainer and let excess moisture drip off to thicken for the dish. To substitute Aleppo pepper, mix 2 teaspoons red pepper (ground) and 2 teaspoons Hungarian pepper. Likewise, you can season the kebab with some paprika, pepper, and salt right before you grill them.

ν Ham Balls   15, 18

Lunch: Servings|4   Prep. Time|**20 minutes**   Cook Time|**0 minutes**
Nut. Content (per serving): Cal|**102**   Fat|**1.8g**   Protein|**15g**   Carbs|**6.7g**

175 grams ham (extra-lean), finely chopped
225 grams quark (fat-free)
4 shallots, finely chopped

Marjoram & chive, finely chopped, adjust to
preference
Tabasco, adjust to preference

1. Mix everything till well blended; form into small balls. Serve.

Baby Back Ribs   17

Entrée: Servings|**2**   Prep. Time|**8 hours**   Cook Time|**3 to 4 minutes per batch**
Nut. Content (per serving): Cal|**454**   Fat|**25.6g**   Protein|**94.2g**   Carbs|**12g**

18-ounce (bottled) barbecue sauce
(vinegar-based)
2 pounds Pork baby back ribs

Cooking spray
Foil (nonstick), large enough line your
baking dish

1. Generously brush your ribs with your BBQ sauce; let marinate for at least 8 hours in the fridge, or leave them overnight for juicier ribs.
2. Line your dish with the foil. If you have no nonstick kind on hand, line with a normal foil and grease with the cooking spray. Put the ribs in the dish; cover with foil to help retain the juices. Bake in a preheated 300F oven for 2 1/2 hours.
NOTES: Alternatively, you can bake the ribs 15 minutes shorter; transfer them to a nonstick foil-lined cookie sheet, brush with more BBQ sauce, and then broil for 15 minutes for juicier ribs. If you want to grill them at the end, bake for 2 hours only and finish cooking on the grill – the meat will become too soft for grilling if you bake them for more than 2 hours.

Iced Tea

Drinks: Servings|**1**   Prep. Time| **Fifteen to Twenty min.**   Cook Time|**0 minutes**
Nut. Content (per serving): Cal|**74**   Fat|**0.1g**   Protein|**0.2g**   Carbs|**21g**

1 cup cold water
1 lemon wedge
1/4 teaspoon tea leaves

2 teaspoon artificial sweeteners (non-fructose based)
2 to 3 ice cubes

1. Boil 1 cup of water in a bowl (stainless steel). Once boiling, turn off the heat; add the tea leaves. Cover the bowl with a lid; let sit for 5 minutes to allow the flavor and the aroma to release. Strain the tea into a cup. Add the sweetener; stir till dissolved. Add the ice, lemon juice, and serve. Garnish with tea if desired.

Oat Bran-Egg White Galette /6

Breakfast: Servings|**1**   Prep. Time **Ten (10) minutes**   Cook Time **Two (2) to three (3) minutes/batch**
Nut. Content (per serving): Cal|**72**   Fat|**4.6g**   Protein|**5.8g**   Carbs|**1.7g**

1 1/2 tablespoon fromage frais (low fat) or quark
1 1/2 to 2 teaspoons oat bran

1 egg white
1 teaspoon olive oil

1. In a bowl, whisk the fromage frais or quark and oat bran with a hand blender till smooth. In a different bowl, whisk the egg white till fluffy. Gently fold the egg white into the bowl with the oat bran mixture – do not whisk the batter at this point or it will reduce the air created by whisking the egg and reduce the fluffiness of the pancake.
2. Turn the heat of your stovetop on to medium heat. Set a frying pan and let warm. Grease the pan with some oil. Ladle 1 spoonful of batter into the pan; cook for 2 to 3 minutes for each side or till both sides are golden brown. Serve hot.
NOTES: For a more savory dish, add some thyme or preferred herbs and spices, such as pepper and paprika.

Vietnamese Beef I5

Dinner: Servings|**2**   Prep. Time|**40 to 45 minutes**   Cook Time|**1 minute**
Nut. Content (per serving): Cal|**280**   Fat|**8.1g**   Protein|**42g**   Carbs|**7g**

1 big thumb ginger, grated
1 tablespoon oyster sauce
2 tablespoons soy sauce
3 drops vegetable oil

4 garlic cloves, crushed
400 grams sirloin steak, sliced into 1-cm chunks
Coriander leaves, to serve

1. Mix the black pepper, ginger, sauces, and beef; let marinate for at least 30 minutes. Sauté the garlic in an oiled frying skillet. Add the beef; stir-fry for 10 to 15 seconds on high heat for medium-rare doneness. Serve garnished with coriander.

Cheesy Omelet 17

Breakfast: Servings|**1**   Prep. Time| **Fifteen to Twenty min.**   Cook Time|**1 minute, 30 seconds**
Nut. Content (per serving): Cal|**495**   Fat|**37.5g**   Protein|**31g**   Carbs|**7.3g**

1 egg (whole)
2 tablespoon olive oil
3 egg whites

4 tablespoon cottage cheese (low-fat), shredded
Pinch pepper
Pinch salt

1. With a blender, whisk the egg whites, egg, pepper, and salt till mixed.
2. Set a skillet over high heat. Once heated, add 2 tablespoons olive oil; spread to coat the bottom of the skillet. When bubbles start to appear, reduce the heat. Quickly add the egg mixture, shaking gently to spread them on the bottom of the skillet evenly.
3. Once the edges of the omelet are cooked, flip and cook for 30 seconds more – do not flatten with the back of a spoon or it will lose its fluffiness. While the omelet is still in the skillet, spread the cheese all over the top. Fold the omelet in half; serve.

Fast Garlic Shrimp 16

Main Dish: Servings|**2**   Prep. Time|**30 to 40 minutes**   Cook Time|**5 minutes**
Nut. Content (per serving): Cal|**876**   Fat|**56.6g**   Protein|**91.9g**   Carbs|**3g**

1 bunch parsley (fresh), chopped
Pinch flakes red pepper
1 teaspoon paprika
1/2 cup olive oil

2 pounds shrimp (large), peeled & deveined
3 tablespoon lemon juice
6 cloves garlic, finely diced
Salt adjust to preference

1. Prepare a large wok or frying pan. Toss the shrimp with the salt, red pepper, paprika, and garlic; let sit aside for 5 to Ten (10) minutes so the shrimp absorb the flavors.
2. Put the olive oil in the wok/pan set over medium heat. Increase the heat at first till small bubbles begin to appear in the oil. Add the shrimp and reduce the heat to medium; stir-fry for 5 minutes or till they are pink. Drizzle with lemon juice; garnish parsley. Serve.

Lemony Chicken Cutlets   17

Entrée: Servings|**4**   Prep. Time|**30 minutes**   Cook Time|**30 to 40 minutes**
Nut. Content (per serving): Cal|**576**   Fat|**43g**   Protein|**33.7g**   Carbs|**28g**

Chicken cutlets:
1 cup oat bran
1 egg
1/2 cup oat bran flour
1/2 cup water
1/2 teaspoon basil
1/2 teaspoon garlic powder
1/2 teaspoon oregano (dried)
1/2 teaspoon parsley, chopped
1/4 cup cottage cheese (low fat), grated
1/4 teaspoon cayenne pepper
1/4 teaspoon pepper

1/4 teaspoon salt
4 chicken breasts, cut into 1/4-inch thin slices
4 tablespoon olive oil

Lemon sauce:
1 tablespoon parsley (fresh), chopped
1/2 teaspoon oregano (dried)
1/4 cup olive oil
1/4 teaspoon black pepper
1/4 teaspoon garlic, finely diced
2 lemons, juice only

1. Sauce: Mix all of the ingredients in a bowl (large) using a fork till well blended.
2. Chicken: Mix the cheese and oat bran in a flat dish. In a different bowl, whisk the water and egg. In a resealable bag, mix the flour, cayenne, pepper, salt, basil, oregano, and garlic. Add the chicken; toss and shake to mix and coat well.
3. Individually, dip the chicken in the egg mixture and then coat with the cheese mixture.
4. Set a skillet on the stovetop. Turn on the flame/heat to medium. Add a couple tablespoons of olive oil in the skillet. Add the chicken and cook till all the sides are golden brown. Serve with the lemon juice.

Yogurt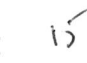

Breakfast: Servings|**1**   Prep. Time|**5 minutes**   Cook Time|**0 minutes**
Nut. Content (per serving): Cal|**126**   Fat|**3.1g**   Protein|**10.5g**   Carbs|**14g**

1 drop of vanilla essence
200 grams yogurt (fat-free)

A couple pinches oat bran
Sweetener, adjust to preference

1. Mix everything till well blended. Serve.

Herbed Omelet *17*

Breakfast: Servings|**1**   Prep. Time|**15 minutes**   Cook Time|**1 minute, 30 seconds**
Nut. Content (per serving): Cal|**424**   Fat|**23.4g**   Protein|**20.3g**   Carbs|**33.2g**

1/4 cup preferred fresh herbs, chopped
1 tablespoon olive oil
1 tablespoon milk (skim)
1 egg white

1 egg
Pepper adjust to preference
Salt adjust to preference

1. In a bowl (medium), whisk the egg white, egg, herbs, pepper, salt, and milk using a blender or with a fork till mixed.
2. Set the frying pan on the stove. Add 1 tablespoon oil; spread on the pan and heat to medium heat. Once small bubbles start to form, add the egg mixture; gently shake the pan to spread it evenly. Once edges of the omelet are cooked, flip, and cook for 30 seconds or more till it fluffs up. Transfer to a plate; serve.

Oat Bran Pancake

Lunch: Servings|**1**   Prep. Time| **Fifteen to Twenty min.**   Cook Time|**4 to 6 minutes per batch**
Nut. Content (per serving): Cal|**448**   Fat|**22g**   Protein|**54g**   Carbs|**11.4g**

1 1/2 tablespoons oat bran
1 1/2 tablespoons quark (fat-free)
175 grams tuna, chicken, smoked salmon, or ham, flaked

2 eggs, separated
Oil, for cooking
Preferred dried herbs, optional

1. Mix the egg yolks, preferred meat, fish, or poultry, a pinch of pepper and salt to preference, herbs, quark, and oat bran. Whisk the egg whites till stiff peaks appear. Fold the egg whites into the yolk mixture.
2. Pour the mixture into a greased, nonstick pan. Cook each side for 2 to 3 minutes or till cooked through.

Herbed Baked Fish *18*

Dinner: Servings|**4**   Prep. Time| **Fifteen to Twenty min.**   Cook Time|**55 minutes**
Nut. Content (per serving): Cal|**392**   Fat|**15g**   Protein|**54.3g**   Carbs|**7g**

3 drops vegetable oil
300 grams fromage frais (fat-free)
4 eggs

5 tablespoons herbs, chopped
800 grams fillets white fish

1. Preheat your oven to 220C. Season the fish and then wrap them with greaseproof paper. Bake for Ten (10) minutes. Lower the temperature of the oven to 180C. Remove the fish and transfer to a blender. Add the herbs, eggs, and fromage frais; blend well.
2. Transfer the fish mixture to a greased baking dish. Put the dish on a larger dish. Fill the larger dish half full with cold water. Bake for 45 minutes or till cooked through.

Lemon Cheesecake

Dessert: Servings|**4**   Prep. Time| **Twenty to Twenty-Five min.**   Cook Time|**40 minutes**
Nut. Content (per serving): Cal|**464**   Fat|**29g**   Protein|**19g**   Carbs|**35.4g**

2 eggs
2 tablespoons corn flour
200 grams cottage cheese
300 grams cream cheese (fat-free)

4 tablespoon fromage frais
4 tablespoon quark
8 tablespoon sweetener
Lemon, grated zest only

1. Preheat your oven to 160C. Except for the cornflour and egg whites, whisk the ingredients till blended, thick, and smooth. In a different bowl, whisk the egg whites till stiff peaks form. Fold in the corn flour. Fold your whisked egg white into your cheese mixture.
2. Transfer the batter into a baking dish; bake for 40 minutes or till risen and golden brown. Let cool completely; serve garnished with the lemon zest.

Beef Rosemary Burgers *p .15*

Lunch: Servings|3   Prep. Time| **Twenty to Twenty-Five min.**   Cook Time| **Fifteen to Twenty min.**
Nut. Content (per serving): Cal|**427**   Fat|**18**   Protein|**55g**   Carbs|**13g**

1 egg, lightly whisked
1 onion, chopped
1 tablespoon Worcestershire sauce (sugar-free)
1 to 2 tablespoons basil or mint, finely chopped

2 garlic cloves, crushed
2 tablespoons plum sauce
2 tablespoons rosemary, finely chopped
750 grams beef (minced)
Salad for serving, optional

1. Mix all of the ingredients, seasoning with pepper and salt to preference. Shape the mixture into patties. Grill till cooked through and both sides are golden brown. Drain excess grease on paper towels.

Fishcake *17*

Dinner: Servings|**1**   Prep. Time|**10 to 15 minutes**   Cook Time|**45 minutes**
Nut. Content (per serving): Cal|**636**   Fat|**33g**   Protein|**57g**   Carbs|**24g**

1 fillet white fish, chopped
1 garlic clove, crushed
1 tablespoon corn flour
3 crabsticks, thinly sliced

3 eggs, separated
6 tablespoon quark (fat-free)
Herbs (chopped), adjust to preference

1. Whisk the egg whites till stiff peaks appear. Fold in the rest of the ingredients. Line a sheet pan with parchment paper. Bake for 45 minutes at 180C or till cooked through.

Coffee Chocolate Meringues

Dessert: Servings|**8**   Prep. Time|**10-15 minutes**   Cook Time|**25 to 30 minutes**
Nut. Content (per serving): Cal|**43**   Fat|**0g**   Protein|**1.3g**   Carbs|**10g**

2 teaspoons cocoa powder
2 teaspoons coffee (very strong)

3 egg whites
6 tablespoons sweetener

1. Preheat your oven to 150C. Whisk the egg whites till very stiff peaks appear. Mix the sweetener and cocoa; sprinkle over the egg whites. Add the coffee; whisk for 30 seconds. Spoon the mixture into small molds set on a sheet pan; bake for 25 to 30 minutes.

Mustard Dill Sauced Salmon Escalopes

Dinner: Servings|**4**   Prep. Time|**15 minutes**   Cook Time|**15 minutes**
Nut. Content (per serving): Cal|**327**   Fat|**15g**   Protein|**44g**   Carbs|**2.5g**

1 tablespoon mustard (mild)
2 shallots, chopped
4 thick (around 200 grams each) salmon pieces

6 teaspoon fromage frais (fat-free)
Dill (finely chopped), adjust to preference
Steamed asparagus, for serving, optional

1. Freeze the salmon for a couple of minutes. Once a bit frozen, cut into 50 grams-thin slices. Gently fry the pieces for 1 minute in a greased nonstick pan. Transfer to a plate and set aside; cover to keep warm.
2. In the same pan, add the shallots and cook till brown. Add the fromage frais and mustard; let simmer for 5 minutes. Return the salmon in the pan. Add the dill and season; cook ti l heated through. Serve with the asparagus.

Chocolate Pannacotta

Dessert: Servings|**1**   Prep. Time|**15 minutes**   Cook Time|**15-20 minutes**
Nut. Content (per serving): Cal|**298**   Fat|**12g**   Protein|**34g**   Carbs|**16g**

5 tablespoons fromage frais (fat-free)
2 leaves gelatin
2 egg yolks

100 ml milk (skimmed)
1 tablespoon protein powder
1 tablespoon cocoa powder

1. Put the gelatin in a bowl. Add cold water and let soften. In a different bowl, mix the protein powder, cocoa powder, and egg yolks till well blended; set aside. Put the milk in a saucepan (small); heat and let come to a boil. While constantly whisking, pour the milk into the egg mixture till well blended.
2. Squeeze excess moisture from the soaked gelatin; add it to the egg mixture. Stir till dissolved completely. Let cool. Add the fromage frais.

Chicken Kebabs

P. 15

Dinner: Servings|**4**   Prep. Time|**2 hours, 20 minutes**   Cook Time|**8 to Ten (10) minutes**
Nut. Content (per serving): Cal|**380**   Fat|**19g**   Protein|**45g**   Carbs|**5.5g**

1 garlic clove, peeled
1 onion, peeled
1 teaspoon garam masala
1/2 tablespoon ground coriander
1/2 tablespoon ground cumin
100 grams yogurt (plain, fat-free)

2 tablespoon coriander, finely chopped
2 tablespoon lemon juice
20 grams ginger, grated
800 grams chicken breasts, sliced into 2-cm cubes
Tzatziki (fat-free), to serve

1. In a blender, puree the garlic and onion; Stir in the coriander, spices, yogurt, lemon juice, and ginger. Transfer to a bowl. Add the chicken; toss to coat well. Marinate in the fridge for 2 hours. Heat your grill to high heat. Thread the chicken onto skewers; cook for 8 to Ten (10) minutes. Serve with the tzatziki.

Is your belly happy yet?

We sincerely hope that you're pleased with the recipes so far. If not, feel free to send us an email at info@limitlessrecipes.com and tell us what we can improve. We get back to every person who reaches out.

If you are enjoying the recipes then you will love the box set below with over 600 delicious and easy to make recipes.

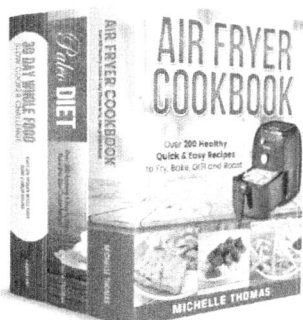

Only sign up for the cookbook box set if you are ready to be absolutely amazed with over 600 proven, delicious and easy to make recipes.

To access the gift page type in www.bit.ly/2Ho82AH or email us at info@limitlessrecipes.com to get the box set delivered to your email.

Limitless Recipes
Like us on Facebook and join our private Facebook group community for more recipes and gifts.
@limitlessrecipes
Follow us on Instagram
Limitless Recipes
Follow us on Pinterest.

Want to be a part of our closed Facebook group?
We are working on building an engaged community discussing recipes and healthy eating in our closed Facebook group. If you would like to be involved in the discussions about cooking, what is working, what is not working and receive information about gifts and promotions, we would be delighted to add you.

Type in Limitless Recipes on Facebook or write us at info@limitlessrecipes.com. Come say hi!

Happy Cooking!

Can we ask you for a quick favor?

We try to write the best cookbooks that we can and a lot of effort goes into writing the cookbook with so many recipes while making sure that the recipes are healthy and fairly easy to make. We sincerely hope you are enjoying the recipes. That being said, reviews really help us A LOT when it comes to putting our names out there and keep us motivated. Competing with big publishing companies is quite hard and reviews really help with making our books more visible.
If you could take one minute to leave a review, we would really appreciate that.

You can leave a review in 3 easy steps:
1. Go to the product page
2. Scroll down and on the left side click 'Write customer review'
3. Write a review and click 'Submit'

Thank you so much. **You are amazing!**

If you feel like we could improve the cookbook please email us at info@limitlessrecipes.com and we'll make sure to get back to you.

Feel free to proceed to the cruise phase recipes, yummy!

CRUISE PHASE (PV)

Crab Stick & Clam Salad

Appetizer: Servings|**1**   Prep. Time|**5 minutes**   Cook Time|**0 minutes**
Nut. Content (per serving): Cal|**249**   Fat|**10.6g**   Protein|**14.4g**   Carbs|**25g**

1 tablespoon capers
1 tablespoon parsley (fresh), chopped
2 crab sticks
6-ounce clams (canned in water), drained

Preferred lettuce, washed & torn into bite-sized pieces
Salt & pepper

1. Put the lettuce in your salad bowl. Break the crab sticks, distribute on top of the greens. Add your clams, parsley, and sprinkle with the capers; season with pepper and salt to preference.

Mustard Chicken & Baked Tomatoes   17

Main Dish: Servings|**2**   Prep. Time|**5 minutes**   Cook Time|**30minutes**
Nut. Content (per serving): Cal|**362**   Fat|**12g**   Protein|**53g**   Carbs|**10g**

2 chicken legs
4 tomatoes (large)
Mustard, as needed

Herbs de Provence or Provencal herbs
Salt & pepper

1. Preheat your oven to 450F. Brush the chicken with mustard; put them in an ovenproof dish and sprinkle with the herb mixture. Put the tomatoes around the chicken. Bake for 30 minutes at 450F.

Creamy Zucchini Soup

Appetizer: Servings|**4**   Prep. Time|**5 minutes**   Cook Time|**25 minutes**
Nut. Content (per serving): Cal|**61**   Fat|**0.4g**   Protein|**3.2g**   Carbs|**13.2g**

1 carrot
1 cube beef stock (low sodium, low-fat)
1 onion (large)

1 tablespoon sour cream (fat-free)
1 turnip
4 zucchini

1. Slice the veggies into bite-sized chunks. Put the veggies in a saucepan. Add enough water just to cover them and the stock cube. Heat and let come to a boil. Once boiling, reduce the heat to a simmer; cook for 20 minutes. Stir in the cream; serve hot.

Salmon & Herbed Oat Bran-Broccoli Tabbouleh 16

Main Dish: Servings|1   Prep. Time **Ten (10) minutes**   Cook Time|**5 minutes**
Nut. Content (per serving): Cal|**588**   Fat|**26.3g**   Protein|**71.6g**   Carbs|**19g**

1 salmon fillet
1/2 lime, grated zest only
1/3 cup florets broccoli
2 spring onions, trimmed & sliced

2 tablespoons oat bran
Handful (small) mint, chopped
Handful (small) parsley, chopped
Salt & pepper, adjust to preference

1. Put the bran in a bowl. Add 2 tablespoons of boiling water; let stand for Ten (10) minutes. Blanch or steam your broccoli in boiling water; drain and refresh under running cold water.
2. Fluff the soaked bran using a fork. Stir in the broccoli, seasoning, lime zest, spring onion, and herbs. Grill the salmon till your desired doneness is achieved. Serve with the tabbouleh. Alternatively, you can flake the salmon and mix with the tabbouleh.

Hibiscus Custard

Dessert: Servings|4   Prep. Time|**30 minutes**   Cook Time|**15 minutes**
Nut. Content (per serving): Cal|**0**   Fat|**0g**   Protein|**0g**   Carbs|**0g**

1 egg
1/4 cup cornstarch (tolerated)
2 cups milk (fat-free)
3 teaspoons tea (dry hibiscus infusion) or 2 tea bags

2 tablespoons Splenda or stevia (granulated sweetener), adjust to preference, preferably organic stevia (Dukan Diet)

1. Heat the milk and let come to boiling. Add your tea; remove from heat, cover, and let sit for Ten (10) minutes to infuse. Pour through a strainer to remove the leaves or remove the bags.
2. In another saucepan, whisk the cornstarch, egg, and sweetener will well mixed. While constantly whisking to prevent the eggs from cooking, add the milk. Set the pan over low heat. While constantly stirring, let the mixture come to a boil. Once boiling, reduce the heat and stir for 3 minutes more. Remove the pan from the heat.
3. Pour the mixture into individual serving dishes or ramekins. Let cool for 1 hour at room temperature. Once cool, refrigerate for 3 hours to chill. Serve chilled.

Barbequed Cod & Wilted Spinach 16

Main Dish: Servings|**2**   Prep. Time **Ten (10) minutes**   Cook Time|**20 minutes**
Nut. Content (per serving): Cal|**383**   Fat|**3.5g**   Protein|**73.7g**   Carbs|**18.1g**

1 bag spinach leaves (baby), washed
1/2 lemon, juice only
14 ounces steak fillets cod

Paprika adjust to preference
Salt & pepper adjust to preference

1. On your grill pan set on your stove or your barbecue; cook the cod for 20 minutes or till the fish is white throughout. While grilling, put the juice of a 1/2 lemon in a frying pan (nonstick, large). Add the spinach; steam cook for a couple of seconds till they start to wilt.
2. Remove the pan from the heat; transfer the spinach to your serving plate and season with pepper and salt to preference. Drizzle with lemon juice and season with paprika. Put the fish on top of the spinach. Serve right away.

Baked Bass

Main Dish: Servings|**2**   Prep. Time **Ten (10) minutes**   Cook Time|**30 minutes**
Nut. Content (per serving): Cal|**342**   Fat|**5.8g**   Protein|**44g**   Carbs|**29g**

1 clove garlic, crushed using your garlic press
1 handful parsley (fresh), finely chopped
1 lemon, cut into slices

2 bass fillets (fresh)
2 onions, peeled & cut into strips
2 tomatoes, sliced into halves
Salt & pepper

1. Preheat your oven to 375F. Spread the onion in a baking dish (ovenproof). Put the fish on top of the onions; surround them with the tomatoes. Put the slices of lemon on the fillets; place any remaining around the fish. Sprinkle the garlic and herbs on the tomatoes; season with pepper and salt.
2. Bake in the preheated oven for 20 to 30 minutes or till the flesh is white throughout, making sure not to overcook them by checking at close to the end of cooking time.

Cinnamon Cake

Dessert: Servings|**6**   Prep. Time|**15minutes**   Cook Time|**25 minutes**
Nut. Content (per serving): Cal|**121**   Fat|**5.5g**   Protein|**13.3g**   Carbs|**14.7g**

1 cup cream cheese (fat-free)
1 tablespoon baking powder
1 tablespoon cornstarch (tolerated)
1 tablespoon wheat bran
1 teaspoon cinnamon
1 teaspoon vanilla extract
1/2 cup milk powder (fat-free)

2 tablespoons milk (fat-free)
2 tablespoons oat bran
2 tablespoons Splenda or stevia (granulated sweetener), adjust to preference, preferably organic stevia (Dukan Diet)
3 eggs, separated

1. Preheat your oven to 325F. Grease an 8x8-inch pan with a couple drops olive oil. Mix the sweetener and the egg yolks. Add the cinnamon, vanilla, cream cheese, baking powder, oat bran, and milk powder; mix till well combined.
2. In a bowl (small), mix the milk (fat-free) and cornstarch till smooth. Add the cornstarch mixture to the egg yolk mixture.
3. In another bowl, whisk the egg whites with an electric beater till soft peaks appear, the ends standing up and then curl under. Gently fold your egg whites with your yolk mixture. Pour the mixture into the prepared pan. Bake for 25 minutes, let cool for 30 minutes and serve.

Smoked Salmon & Cabbage Salad   17

Appetizer: Servings|**6**   Prep. Time|**15 minutes**   Cook Time|**0 minutes**
Nut. Content (per serving): Cal|**47**   Fat|**1g**   Protein|**3.5g**   Carbs|**7.5g**

1/2 head cabbage (green), grated or chopped
1/2 head cabbage (red), grated or chopped

2 shallots, finely sliced
3 smoked salmon slices, sliced into thin strips

1. Toss the shallots and cabbage. Gently toss in the salmon.

Curry Creamy Beets

Appetizer: Servings|**2**   Prep. Time|**30 minutes**   Cook Time|**0 minutes**
Nut. Content (per serving): Cal|**59**   Fat|**0.5g**   Protein|**3.5g**   Carbs|**11.3g**

1 egg white
2 tablespoon sour cream (fat-free)
2 teaspoon curry powder

8 ounces (canned) beets
Salt

1. Blend the beets in your blender till smooth. In a bowl, whisk the curry powder, a pinch of salt, egg white, and cream till mixed. Divide the beet puree between serving dishes. Divide the cream and spread on top of the beets. Refrigerate for 1 hour or till chilled before serving.

Easy Stir-Fry Seafood

Main Dish: Servings|**4**   Prep. Time|**20 minutes**   Cook Time **Ten (10) minutes**
Nut. Content (per serving): Cal|**164**   Fat|**5.1g**   Protein|**21g**   Carbs|**9g**

1 ounce shiitake mushrooms (dried) or 1
1/2 cups mushrooms (fresh)
1 tablespoon soy sauce (low sodium)
1 teaspoon olive oil, divided (tolerated)
1/2 cup chicken broth (low sodium, fat-free)
1/2 pound sea scallops, halved, or bay
scallops

1/4 cup green onions, thinly sliced
1/4 pound raw shrimp (medium), peeled &
deveined
2 cloves garlic, minced
2 cups green beans
2 packs Shirataki rice (Dukan Diet)
4 1/2 teaspoons cornstarch (tolerated)

1. Prepare the shirataki rice following the package directions; set aside.
2. Put the mushrooms in a bowl (small). Cover with boiling water; let sit for 20 minutes to soak and soften. Drain and squeeze out excess water. Discard the stems and slice the caps.
3. In a different bowl (small), mix the cornstarch, soy sauce, and broth till smooth; set aside. In a wok or nonstick skillet, heat 1/2 teaspoon of oil on medium heat. Add the shrimp, scallops, and garlic, stir-fry for 3 minutes or till the seafood is opaque. Transfer to a bowl; set aside.
4. Add the remaining 1/2 teaspoon of oil in the wok/skillet. Add the green beans and mushrooms; stir-fry for 3 minutes or till the beans are tender-crisp. Stir the broth mixture; add to the wok; stir-fry for 2 minutes or till the sauce is thick. Add the seafood mixture, along with any juices in the wok; cook till warmed through. Sprinkle with the green onions. Serve plated with the shirataki rice.

Baked Eggplant

Appetizer: Servings|**1**   Prep. Time **Ten (10) minutes**   Cook Time|**45 to 60 minutes**
Nut. Content (per serving): Cal|**141**   Fat|**1g**   Protein|**5.6g**   Carbs|**33.2g**

1 clove garlic, crushed using your garlic
press

1 eggplant
Pinch powdered coriander

1. Preheat your oven to 400F. Slice the stem of your eggplant. Pierce it a couple of times using s fork to prevent it from bursting while it cooks. Put it on a sheet pan; bake for 45 to 60 minutes or till the skin is blanched and the meat is softened.
2. Once the eggplant is cooked, remove from the skin. Peel off the burnt skin. Shop the flesh into bite-sized chunks. Add the coriander and garlic; mix well. Chill and serve.

Baked Monkfish and Tomato Loaf *A*

Main Dish: Servings|6   Prep. Time|**20 minutes**   Cook Time|**30 minutes**
Nut. Content (per serving): Cal|**117**   Fat|**3.7g**   Protein|**17.7g**   Carbs|**2.9g**

1 cube chicken stock
1 head lettuce, rinsed
1 pound monkfish (fresh)
1 tablespoon "persillade" (crushed garlic & chopped parsley)

1/4 cup tomato sauce
3 eggs
Balsamic vinegar
Salt & pepper

1. In a saucepan with boiling water, dissolve the stock cube. Add the fish; cook for 15 minutes. Preheat your oven to 350F. Remove the fish from the stock; strain to drain. Slice them into 1-inch chunks; set aside.
2. Mix the tomato sauce and eggs; season with pepper and salt to preference. Add the persillade; stir to mix well. Grease a loaf pan with a couple drops of olive oil. Set your fish on your pan. Pour the egg mixture on the top of the fish evenly.
3. Bake for 30 minutes. If the topping browns to0 quickly, cover the pan with aluminum foil for the rest of the cooking time. Remove the pan from the oven; let rest for 15 minutes. Carefully remove the fish from the pan by running a butter knife around the edges to dislodge it. Invert onto a plate.
4. Tear the lettuce into bite-sized pieces; divide between 6 serving plates. Evenly slice the loaf into 6 portions. Place 1 slice on top of each lettuce bed. Drizzle with balsamic vinegar. Serve.

Cauliflower Soup

Appetizer: Servings|4   Prep. Time|**45 minutes**   Cook Time|**45 to 55 minutes**
Nut. Content (per serving): Cal|**86**   Fat|**0.6g**   Protein|**6.6g**   Carbs|**16g**

1 cup mushrooms, steamed
1 tablespoon Agar-Agar powder
1 teaspoon cumin powder
2 cups milk (fat-free)
8 ounces cauliflower, steamed

Flakes Maldon salt (or any Salt (sea) crystals)
Sichuan pepper, or Timur or Nepal or pepper, in Oriental stores

1. Except for the mushrooms, mix the rest of the ingredients will well-combined. Transfer the mixture into a casserole (large); let come to a boil. Once boiling, lower the heat; simmer for 30 minutes. Transfer the mixture to a dish (small); sprinkle with the mushrooms. Refrigerate for at least 4 hours to chill before serving.

Baked Provencal Cod 17

Main Dish: Servings|4   Prep. Time|**25 minutes**   Cook Time|**15 minutes**
Nut. Content (per serving): Cal|**194**   Fat|**3g**   Protein|**28g**   Carbs|**16g**

1 pound (4-ounce each) cod fillets (skinless)
2 garlic cloves, thinly sliced
2 onions, peeled &thinly sliced
3 basil leaves
8 slices ham (extra-lean)
8 tomatoes, stems removed

Salt & black pepper (freshly ground, adjust to preference

Materials:
4 pieces (2-cup) ramekins

1. Preheat your oven to 475F. Put 1 slice of ham into each ramekin. Fill a pot with water and let come to a boil. Add the tomatoes; poach for 30 seconds. Remove immediately. Peel the skins off from the tomatoes, remove the seeds, and slice. Divide the tomatoes between the ramekins, topping on the ham; season with salt to preference. Top with the onion and then the garlic.
2. Wrap the cod fillets with the remaining ham. Put each ham-wrapped fish on top of each dish; season with pepper & salt to preference. Bake for 15 minutes. Once cooked, remove the ramekins from the oven; season with more black pepper to preference. Garnish with the basil leaves; serve.

Shrimp-Stuffed Peppers 17

Appetizer: Servings|2   Prep. Time|**20 minutes**   Cook Time|**30 minutes**
Nut. Content (per serving): Cal|**165**   Fat|**1g**   Protein|**31g**   Carbs|**10g**

10 ounces shrimp (large), cooked & peeled
2 cloves garlic, crushed using your garlic press
Salt (sea) & pepper adjust to preference

2 preferred color (green, red, or yellow) bell peppers of your choice (large)
2 tomatoes, peeled, seeds removed, & diced

1. Preheat your oven to 350F. Gently fry your shrimp and garlic in a frying pan (nonstick) for 2 to 3 minutes. Add the tomatoes, season with pepper and salt to preference, and simmer for 2 to 3 minutes. Remove the pan from heat.
2. Cut the tops off from the bell peppers. Remove the seeds and ribs; discard. Stuff each pepper with the shrimp mixture; bake for 30 minutes. Serve right away.

Coffee Cream Rum Cakes

Dessert: Servings|**2**   Prep. Time **Ten (10) minutes**   Cook Time|**20 minutes**
Nut. Content (per serving): Cal|**336**   Fat|**10g**   Protein|**10g**   Carbs|**55g**

Batter:
1 tablespoon baking powder
1 tablespoon cornstarch (tolerated)
1 tablespoon wheat bran
1/3 cup milk (fat-free)
2 egg yolks
2 tablespoons oat bran
2 tablespoons Splenda or stevia (granulated sweetener), adjust to preference, preferably organic stevia (Dukan Diet)

Coffee syrup:
1 cup espresso (strongly brewed)
1/2 teaspoon white rum (tolerated)
1/4 cup water
3 tablespoons Splenda or stevia (granulated sweetener), adjust to preference, preferably organic stevia (Dukan Diet)

Custard:
1 tablespoon cornstarch (tolerated)
1 tablespoon Splenda or stevia (granulated sweetener), adjust to preference, preferably organic stevia (Dukan Diet)
1 tablespoon water, at room temperature or cooler
1 teaspoon cocoa powder (unsweetened), such as Cocoa Powder (Dukan Diet), organic (tolerated)
1 teaspoon gelatin powder (unflavored)
1 teaspoon strong coffee or instant coffee granules, brewed
1 teaspoon white rum (tolerated)
1/4 cup milk (fat-free)
2 egg yolks

Materials:
2 pieces ovenproof ramekins or muffin cups

1. Preheat your oven to 350F. Grease the ramekins/cups with a couple drops olive oil.
2. Batter: Mix the sweetener and yolks. Add the milk, baking powder, cornstarch, wheat bran, and oat bran; mix well. With your electric mixer, whisk the egg whites till stiff peaks appear, the tips standing up.
3. Gently fold the egg whites into the egg yolk mixture. Divide the mixture between the ramekins; bake for 20 minutes. Once cooked, transfer to a cooling rack; let cool for 5 minutes before removing from the containers.
4. Custard: Put the water in a microwavable bowl. Sprinkle the gelatin in the water; stir to distribute. Let sit for 1 minute and microwave for 30 to 40 seconds; stir to dissolve the gelatin.
5. Put the milk in a saucepan; let come to a boil. While the milk is heating up, mix the rum, cocoa powder, coffee, cornstarch, sweetener, and 2 eggs in a bowl. Once your milk reaches boiling, remove your pan from the flame. Add the gelatin mixture; stir well to mix.
6. While constantly mixing the milk mixture, add the egg mixture gradually in the saucepan to prevent the eggs from cooking. Once all the eggs are mixed in, reduce the heat to low. Constantly stir the mixture till thick. Watch carefully and make sure the custard does not come to a boil. Once creamy, remove the saucepan from the heat; refrigerate to cool.

7. Rum syrup: Mix all of the ingredients in a saucepan; heat on the stovetop over low heat till dissolved and mixed. Transfer the cakes into individual serving platters; pour the syrup on top and allow the cake to absorb the syrup for a few seconds. Top with a spoonful of custard. Serve.

Yule Log I

Dessert: Servings|**6**   Prep. Time|**30 minutes**   Cook Time|**5 minutes**
Nut. Content (per serving): Cal|**202**   Fat|**6.6g**   Protein|**7.7g**   Carbs|**26.2g**

5 fluid ounces milk (fat-free)
1/2 packet gelatin (unflavored)
1 egg (whole)
3 eggs, separated
3 tablespoons cornstarch (tolerated), divided
1/2 packet yeast

1 teaspoon vanilla flavoring
7 tablespoons sweetener zero-calorie, such as stevia (organic, Dukan Diet) or Splenda, adjust to preference, divided
1 teaspoon chocolate flavoring
1 teaspoon cocoa (low-fat), such as Cocoa Powder (organic, Dukan Diet), tolerated

1. Pastry cream: Put the milk in a saucepan; heat it and let come to a boil.
2. Soften the gelatin with some warm water. Break the whole egg in a bowl, add the chocolate flavoring, 2 tablespoons sweetener, and 1 teaspoon cornstarch; mix till smooth.
3. Add the hot milk; stir to mix. Return the mixture in the saucepan and heat over low heat; stir till the mixture is thick. Remove the pan from the heat. Stir in the gelatin mixture till mixed. Refrigerate till chilled.
4. Sponge: Mix the 3 yolks with the vanilla flavoring, 5 tablespoons sweetener, and cornstarch till well combined. Preheat the oven to 320F. Whisk the egg whites, till stiff peaks appear. Carefully fold your egg white with your yolk mixture.
5. Spread the batter into a 10x12-inch nonstick baking dish. Put on the center rack of your; bake for five (5) minutes. Once baked, remove from the oven. Carefully lift the sponge from the dish to prevent breaking it.
6. Carefully spread the cream over 3/4 of the sponge, and then roll widthwise to push the excess cream to cover the bare side. Refrigerate and let cool for at least 2 hours to chill. Sprinkle with the cocoa just before serving.

Beetroot & Egg Salad

Appetizer: Servings|**1**   Prep. Time|**5 minutes**   Cook Time|**0 minutes**
Nut. Content (per serving): Cal|**259**   Fat|**10g**   Protein|**11g**   Carbs|**33.6g**

1 beetroot
1 egg (hard-boiled)
Salt & pepper

Balsamic vinegar or preferred vinaigrette (oil-free)

1. Slice the beetroot. Put the slices in a serving platter. Crush the yolks of the egg; sprinkle on top of the beetroot. Drizzle with a splash of vinegar or vinaigrette; season with pepper and salt to preference.

Sweet Squash Flan w/ Caramel Coulis

Dessert: Servings|6   Prep. Time|**20 minutes**   Cook Time|**80 minutes**
Nut. Content (per serving): Cal|**250**   Fat|**6.8g**   Protein|**9.8g**   Carbs|**41g**

1 pound nutmeg or butternut squash
1 teaspoon cornstarch (tolerated)
1/2 teaspoon cinnamon
1/4 teaspoon ginger powder
2 cups milk (fat-free)
2 tablespoons oat bran, such as Oat bran (organic, Dukan Diet)
4 eggs, beaten
4 tablespoons Splenda or stevia (granulated sweetener), adjust to preference, preferably organic stevia (Dukan Diet)
Pinch salt

1/4 orange, zest only

Caramel coulis:
1 teaspoon caramel extract (or 1/2 teaspoon maple extract or 1 tablespoon caramel flavor (sugar-free) syrup, such as Torani)
1 teaspoon gelatin powder
1/2 cup Splenda or stevia (granulated sweetener), adjust to preference, preferably organic stevia (Dukan Diet)
1/4 cup water

1. Preheat your oven to 400F. Grease 6 muffin cups or ramekins with cooking spray (nonstick). Slice the squash flesh into 2-inch chunks. Put the milk and squash into a saucepan; let come to a simmer for 20 minutes, uncovered.
2. In a different pan with boiling water, add the orange zest. After 3 boiling for 3 minutes, drain and chop to smaller pieces.
3. Mash the squash mixture using a vegetable mill or a potato ricer. Add the salt, eggs, oat bran, cornstarch, orange zest, cinnamon, ginger, and sweetener; mix well.
4. Pour the mixture into your greased ramekins. Put them in an ovenproof pan or cookie sheet filled halfway with water for the bain-marie or water bath. Cook in the oven for 1 hour. When cooked, let cool completely before removing from the ramekins.
5. Put the water in a microwavable bowl. Sprinkle the gelatin inside; stir to distribute and let sit for 1 minute. Microwave for 30 to 40 seconds; stir till the gelatin is dissolved. Add the caramel flavoring and sweetener; stir to dissolve. Pour the mixture over the flan. Chill in your fridge for a minimum of 2 hours; serve.

After-Eight Flan

Dessert: Servings|6   Prep. Time **Ten (10) minutes**   Cook Time|**20minutes**
Nut. Content (per serving): Cal|**143**   Fat|**8.3g**   Protein|**9.7g**   Carbs|**6g**

1 1/2 cups milk (fat-free)
1 tablespoon cocoa powder (unsweetened),
such as Cocoa Powder (organic, Dukan
Diet), tolerated
1 tablespoon cornstarch (tolerated)

1 vanilla pod
5 eggs
A couple drops peppermint extract
Pinch nutmeg powder

1. Preheat your oven to 325F. Whisk the eggs. Put the vanilla pod and milk in a saucepan; heat it up but do let it come to a boil. While constantly stirring, gently and gradually add the hot warm milk into the beaten eggs till mixed. Add the nutmeg, peppermint extract, and cornstarch.
2. Divide the mixture between 6 ramekins; cook in the oven for Fifteen to Twenty min.. Refrigerate for at least 4 hours to chill. Sprinkle with the chocolate powder before serving.

Berry Tarts

Dessert: Servings|4   Prep. Time **Ten (10) minutes**   Cook Time|**60 minutes**
Nut. Content (per serving): Cal|**87**   Fat|**1.3g**   Protein|**3.5g**   Carbs|**17.4g**

1 teaspoon baking powder
1/2 cup yogurt (plain, fat-free)
1/2 teaspoon strawberry or raspberry
extract
2 egg whites
2 tablespoons cornstarch (tolerated)

2 tablespoons oat bran
2 teaspoons wheat bran
3 tablespoons granulated sweetener
(Splenda) or 1/3 teaspoon stevia, preferably
organic (Dukan Diet)

1. Preheat your oven (convection) to 300F. Grease 4 muffin cup tins with a couple drops of your olive oil.
2. With an electric beater, whisk the egg whites till soft peaks appear, the tips standing up and curling under. Add the flavor extract, oat bran, wheat bran, cornstarch, yogurt, and sweetener; stir till just mixed.
3. Bake for 1 hour. Once done, remove from your oven; let cool. Chill in your fridge for a minimum of 2 hours; serve.

Herbed Cod Packets 18

Main Dish: Servings|4   Prep. Time|**15 minutes**   Cook Time|**15 minutes**
Nut. Content (per serving): Cal|**113**   Fat|**1.9g**   Protein|**19g**   Carbs|**5.4g**

1 teaspoon olive oil
1/2 lemon, juice only
2 bell peppers (1 red, 1 yellow), sliced into small chunks
4 cod fillets
4 coriander sprigs, washed, dried, & roughly chopped

4 parsley sprigs, washed, dried, & roughly chopped
4 shallots, peeled & thinly sliced
4 tarragon sprigs, washed, dried, & roughly chopped
Salt & pepper

1. Heat your oil in a pan (nonstick). Once heated, add the shallots, cook for 4 minutes or till starting to brown. Remove from heat. Add the herbs; stir to mix well.
2. Cut 4 pieces of rectangle-shaped parchment paper. Put 1 cod on the middle of each paper; season the fillets with pepper and salt to preference. Divide the shallot mixture between them, placing on top of the fish; drizzle each with lemon juice. Securely close the parchment paper, making packets.
3. Put the packets in a sheet pan. Bake in a preheated 425F oven for Ten (10) minutes. Once cooked, remove from the oven; let sit for 5 minutes. Serve the peppers with the parcels.

Shrimp Green Chili 18

Main Dish: Servings|4   Prep. Time **Ten (10) minutes**   Cook Time|**5 minutes**
Nut. Content (per serving): Cal|**119**   Fat|**1g**   Protein|**24.2g**   Carbs|**4.8g**

1 garlic clove, crushed
1 green chili (fresh), seeds removed & chopped
1 lime, juice only

2 tablespoons cilantro (fresh), chopped
1 pound (around 32) shrimps (large)
4 tomatoes, stems removed
Salt

1. Fill a pot (medium) with water, heat and let come to a boil. Once boiling, add the tomatoes; poach for 30 seconds. Remove the tomatoes from the pot. Peel the skin off, remove the seeds, and dice the flesh.
2. In a bowl (medium), mix the garlic, lime juice, cilantro, cilantro, chili, tomatoes, and salt to preference.
3. Fill a steamer (large) halfway full with water; heat and let come to a simmer. Put the shrimp on the steamer basket. Steam for 3 minutes or till they are opaque and pink. Mix the tomato mixture and shrimp. Serve while warm or chill before serving.

Leek-y Creole Shrimp

Main Dish: Servings|**2**   Prep. Time|**30 minutes**   Cook Time **Ten (10) minutes**
Nut. Content (per serving): Cal|**174**   Fat|**4g**   Protein|**6g**   Carbs|**30.4g**

Shrimp:
1/8 teaspoon olive oil
3/4 cup yogurt (Greek, fat-free)
4 leeks (large)
40 to 60 shrimps (peeled, cleaned & frozen or raw)
Caribbean curry powder (a mixture of poppy, cumin, coriander, cloves, mustard seeds, ground turmeric & ginger)

Parsley vinaigrette, recipe below
Salt & pepper

Parsley vinaigrette:
1 tablespoon vinegar (red wine)
1/8 teaspoon olive oil (extra-virgin)
2 tablespoons parsley (flat-leaf, fresh), roughly chopped
3/4 tablespoon shallots, finely diced

1. Parsley vinaigrette: Put the vinegar and shallots in a mixing bowl (medium). While constantly whisking, add the olive oil. Add the parsley and season with pepper and salt to preference.
2. Shrimp: Clean the leeks. Add water and heat. Once it starts to steam, turn off heat. Let sit fo8 minutes before draining. Separate the white and green parts. Set the green parts aside as a garnish.
3. If using raw shrimps, then clean them. Coat a frying pan (nonstick) with 1/8 teaspoon olive oil. Heat and fry the shrimp, seasoning with pepper and salt in the process. Add the yogurt; stir to mix. Add the curry powder, adjusting to preference.
4. In another frying pan; stir-fry the leeks with olive oil, seasoning with pepper, salt, and the parsley vinaigrette. Arrange the leeks and shrimp on a serving plate. Serve hot.

Crab Meat Cucumber Cups

Appetizer: Servings|**4**   Prep. Time|**15 minutes**   Cook Time|**0 minutes**
Nut. Content (per serving): Cal|**251**   Fat|**6.5g**   Protein|**25g**   Carbs|**26g**

1 cucumber
2 tablespoons preferred mixed herbs
4 crab sticks, sliced
4 ounces sour cream (fat-free)
4 tablespoons chives, chopped

5 to 6 ounces crab meat (fresh)
8 asparagus sticks, to decorate
Lemon flavoring
Salt & pepper

1. Wash the cucumbers and trim off the ends. Using your vegetable peeler, peel it lengthwise in an alternative skin-on, skin-off manner. Slice the cucumber into 8 portions. Scoop out the center flesh from each portion, leaving a 1/2-cm thick bottom and borders to form a cup.
2. Drain the crab meat; flake them using a fork. Mix the flaked crab meat with a couple drops lemon flavoring, chives. Herbs, and sour cream, seasoning with pepper and salt to preference.
3. Divide the crab mixture between the cucumber cups set on a serving platter. Sprinkle the top with chives and garnish with crab sticks. Decorate with asparagus spears and whole crab sticks.

Seafood Skewers & Vegetable Medley   /7

Main Dish: Servings|**2 to 4**   Prep. Time|**30 minutes**   Cook Time|**30 minutes**
Nut. Content (per 4 servings): Cal|350   Fat|**6g**   Protein|**40g**   Carbs|**35g**

For 6 skewers:
1 teaspoon curry powder
18 cherry tomatoes
18 shrimps
36 to 40 scallops
5 tablespoons cream (fat-free)
Parsley vinaigrette, recipe below
Salt (sea) & pepper

Parsley vinaigrette:
1 tablespoon vinegar (red wine)
1/8 teaspoon olive oil (extra-virgin)
2 tablespoons parsley (flat-leaf, fresh),
roughly chopped
3/4 tablespoon shallots, finely diced

Vegetable medley:
1 bag (10 to 12 ounces) frozen mixed
vegetables
2 shallots
1 clove garlic, finely chopped
1 teaspoon curry powder
1/2 teaspoon powdered ginger
1 cup tomato puree (or a mixture of 1/2 cup
tomato paste & 1/2 cup water)
3/4 cup yogurt (Greek, plain, fat-free)
2 tablespoons soy sauce (low-sodium)
1 teaspoon cornstarch (tolerated)
Salt (sea)& pepper
Olive oil

1. Parsley vinaigrette: Put the vinegar and shallots in a mixing bowl (medium). While constantly whisking, add the olive oil. Mix in the parsley and season with pepper and salt to preference. Divide into 2 portions.

2. Vegetable medley: Grease a pan (nonstick) with olive oil. Add the veggies, garlic, and shallots; stir-fry for Ten (10) minutes. Season with pepper, salt, the spices, and 1/2 of the parsley vinaigrette. Add 1 cup water, soy sauce, and tomato puree. Reduce the heat; let simmer for 30 minutes. In a bowl (small), mix the yogurt and cornstarch. Add to the veggies, stir to mix and thicken.

3. Seafood skewers: Heat a pan (nonstick) with olive oil. Just before cooking, season scallops with pepper and salt; fry till just cooked. Add the rest of the parsley vinaigrette, curry powder, sour cream till well combined. Add the tomatoes; let simmer for a couple of minutes. Remove from heat.

4. Skewer the scallops, shrimp, and tomatoes between 6 kebab sticks. Grill or bake. If you have a frying pan that is long, fry them in the pan.

Vegetable & Marinated Beef Kebabs

Main Dish: Servings|**2**   Prep. Time|**25 minutes**   Cook Time|**20 minutes**
Nut. Content (per serving): Cal|**374**   Fat|**14.4g**   Protein|**46g**   Carbs|**14g**

Marinade:
1 tablespoon soy sauce (low sodium)
1 teaspoon lemon juice
1 teaspoon Splenda or stevia (organic,
Dukan Diet), adjust to preference
Pinch cayenne pepper
Pinch ginger powder

Material:
6 kebab skewers (wooden), soaked for 15
minutes in water & coated with a couple
drops olive oil

Kebabs:
1 bell pepper (yellow, green, or red), seeds
removed & sliced into large chunks
10 ounces beef tenderloin or top sirloin
(lean), sliced into large chunks
2 shiitake or porcini mushrooms (large),
rinsed & sliced into large chunks
6 cherry tomatoes

1. In a mixing bowl (large), mix all the marinade ingredients. Add the beef chunks; stir and toss to coat well. Marinate in the fridge for 4 hours, stirring every hour.
2. Preheat your oven to 350F. In alternating order, skewer the veggies and beef chunks onto the kebab sticks. Place the kebabs an ovenproof, nonstick dish; cook for 20 minutes, flipping often to cook all sides evenly.

Hot Cocoa

Drinks: Servings|**1**   Prep. Time|**5 minutes**   Cook Time| **Fifteen to Twenty min.**
Nut. Content (per serving): Cal|**177**   Fat|**2g**   Protein|**10.4g**   Carbs|**34.2g**

1 1/2 tablespoons sweetener
1 cup milk (skimmed)
1/4 teaspoon vanilla extract

2 tablespoons cocoa powder
(unsweetened)
Pinch salt

1. Blend 2 tablespoons milk, vanilla extract, salt, and cocoa powder in a saucepan set on medium flame. Once well combined, add the rest of the milk; stir and heat till desired hotness is achieved. Add sweetener to preference. Serve in your favorite mug.
NOTES: If you want to serve this cold, just mix everything in your blender. Serve with ice cubes.

Seared Tuna & Arugula 16 , 18

Appetizer: Servings|**6**   Prep. Time|**20 minutes**   Cook Time|**5 minutes**
Nut. Content (per serving): Cal|**88**   Fat|**1.6g**   Protein|**16.2g**   Carbs|**3.8g**

1 pound tuna steak (fresh)
1 tablespoon balsamic vinegar
1 tablespoon mustard
1 tablespoon wheat bran
1/2 pounds arugula

1/2 teaspoon olive oil
2 tablespoons oat bran, preferably oat bran
(organic, Dukan Diet)
Salt & pepper

1. Wash the arugula and dry them. Divide between 6 serving bowls; set aside.
2. Dressing: In a mixing bowl, mix the oil, vinegar, mustard, pepper, and salt to preference till well combined; set aside.
3. Mix the wheat bran and oat bran in a bowl (small); set aside.
4. Cut the tuna into 1-inch thick strips. Roll each strip in the bran mixture to coat well. Heat a frying pan (nonstick); add the oil. Once heated, fry the tuna for 3 to 4 minutes or till desired doneness is achieved. Let the seared tuna cool.
5. To serve, dress the arugula with the dressing. Put tuna strips on top of them.

Cheesy Spinach Muffins 16

Main Dish/Snack: Servings|**2**   Prep. Time|**20 minutes**   Cook Time|**30 minutes**
Nut. Content (per 2 servings): Cal|**222**   Fat|**12g**   Protein|**16.2g**   Carbs|**22g**

1 egg (whole), beaten
1/2 teaspoon baking powder
2 tablespoons cream cheese (nonfat),
fromage frais or quark
2 tablespoons wheat bran (Dukan Diet)

4 tablespoons milk powder (skimmed)
4 tablespoons oat bran (Dukan D et)
500 grams of spinach leaves (frozen)
Pinch salt & pepper

1. Preheat your oven to 180C. Put the spinach in a frying pan. Turn the heat on to low heat. Let the spinach thaw for Ten (10) minutes or till softened. Transfer to a blender, process till shredded, and squeeze to drain moisture; set aside.
2. In a bowl, mix the beaten egg, salt, baking powder, milk powder, wheat bran, oat bran, and spinach. Divide the mixture between silicone muffin cups or a loaf pan, filling only half full. Put a dollop of cream cheese into each mold and top with the remaining egg mixture.
3. Bake in the oven for 20 minutes or till golden and puffed. Once cooked, remove from the oven; let stand for 5 minutes. Remove from the molds before serving. Serve with a side of salad as a main dish or plainly as a snack.

Yule Log II

Dessert: Servings|6   Prep. Time|**30 minutes**   Cook Time|**15 minutes**
Nut. Content (per serving): Cal|**508**   Fat|**31g**   Protein|**15.5g**   Carbs|**46g**

1 heaping tablespoon agar-agar (Dukan) or
4 sheets gelatin
1 sachet yeast
1/2 cup & 300 ml milk (skimmed), divided
17 tablespoons granulated sweetener
(Splenda), divided
2 teaspoons dark chocolate flavoring
2 teaspoons of vanilla flavoring

2 teaspoons orange blossom water,
optional
6 tablespoons cornflour, divided
6 teaspoons cocoa (reduced-fat, Dukan)
7 tablespoons powdered milk (skim)
8 eggs, divided
Granulated sweetener (Splenda)
Pinch salt

1. Cream filling: Put the 300 ml milk in a saucepan; heat on low heat. If using gelatin sheets instead of agar-agar, soak them in a bit of cold water and let sit; drain before using. In a bowl (large), mix 2 whole eggs, chocolate flavoring, 4 teaspoons sweetener, and 2 tablespoons cornflour till the mixture is smooth.

2. While constantly stirring, gradually add the heated milk till the mixture is thick. Add the drained gelatin sheets or agar-agar; stir to mix and set aside in the fridge while making the sponge cake.

3. Sponge cake: Preheat your oven to 180C. Separate the remaining eggs into yolks and whites. Mix the yolks with the vanilla flavoring, orange blossom water, 10 tablespoons sweetener, 4 tablespoons cornflour, and yeast.

4. In a different bowl, whisk the egg whites with 1 pinch salt till stiff peaks appear. Gently fold the egg white into the yolk mixture – do not stir too briskly. Line a rimmed sheet pan with parchment paper. Spread the dough in the pan into 1-cm thick rectangular shape using a rolling pin. Bake for 8 to Ten (10) minutes in the oven.

5. Once cooked, remove the cake from the oven; let cool. Remove the cake from the parchment paper, making sure not the tear/break the cake. Transfer the sponge cake in a moist clean towel. Spread a layer of cream filling across the top. Roll the cake lengthwise into a log.

6. Frosting: Mix the milk powder, 3 teaspoons sweetener, and the cocoa. Gradually add the liquid milk till your create a creamy, spreadable frosting. Cover the log with the frosting and dust with cocoa powder. Refrigerate for at least 4 hours to chill and serve. Can be served for the Consolidation and Stabilization Phases.

Goji Berry Caramel Jam

Breakfast/Dessert: Servings|0   Prep. Time|**5 minutes**   Cook Time **Ten (10) minutes**
Nut. Content (per 1 tbsp.): Cal|**9**   Fat|**0g**   Protein|**0g**   Carbs|**2.2g**

1 tablespoon liquid sweetener, adjust to preference
1 teaspoon agar-agar (Dukan)
1 teaspoon lemon juice

2 teaspoons strawberry flavoring (Dukan)
5 tablespoons goji berries
Water, as needed to cover the berries)

1. Put the berries in a saucepan (nonstick, small). Add just enough water to cover them. Add the lemon juice and the sweetener. Heat and let come to a boil. Once boiling, add the agar-agar; stir to mix well. Simmer for 7 minutes while constantly stirring to prevent from sticking to the pan and burning, adding a bit of water as needed.
2. The jam is ready when the berries have fattened and caramelized. Transfer the jam in mason jars with tight lids. Store for a maximum of 4 days in your fridge. This jam makes a great topping for your pancakes. Can be served for this phase and onwards.

Pumpkin Muffins 17 , 18

Breakfast: Servings|**6**   Prep. Time|**30 minutes**   Cook Time|**40 minutes**
Nut. Content (per serving): Cal|**318**   Fat|**20.4g**   Protein|**16.6g**   Carbs|**24.4g**

1 sachet baking powder
1 teaspoon ground cinnamon
2 eggs
2 teaspoons white rum flavoring (Dukan)
200 grams pumpkin (raw weight)

3 tablespoons milk powder (skimmed)
4 tablespoons cream cheese (low-fat, 0%)
6 tablespoons sweetener
9 tablespoons oat bran
Pinch nutmeg

1. With a spoon (large), clean your pumpkin, removing the rind. Slice the flesh into small chunks. Steam for Ten (10) minutes or put in a metal sheet pan and bake for 20 minutes at 200C. Once cooked, transfer to a blender and puree till smooth.
2. In a bowl, mix the milk powder, cinnamon, nutmeg, baking powder, and oat bran till well combined. Add the flavoring, eggs, cheese, sweetener, and pureed pumpkin; mix well. Transfer the mixture to muffin cups, filling each mold 2/3full. Bake for 40 minutes in a preheated 180C oven.

Cream of Mushroom Sauce

Appetizer: Servings|**2 to 4**   Prep. Time|**15 minutes**   Cook Time|**10 to 15 minutes**
Nut. Content (per 2 servings): Cal|**188**   Fat|**16.4g**   Protein|**5.2g**   Carbs|**5.3g**

1 tablespoon olive oil
100 ml cream (low fat)
2 cups mushrooms, sliced

2 tablespoon cream cheese (low fat)
Pepper, adjust to preference
Salt, adjust to preference

1. Heat your saucepan to medium heat. Add the olive oil. Once the oil starts to bubble, add the mushrooms; sauté for 5 to 6 minutes or till their moisture evaporates and they are dry.
2. Add the cheese; stir for 2 minutes. Add the cream and season with pepper and salt to preference. Remove from the heat and serve. You can serve this as an appetizer, a dipping sauce, or a pair for your favorite grilled beef and chicken recipe.

Bacon Scrambled Egg   17

Breakfast: Servings|**2**   Prep. Time **Ten (10) minutes**   Cook Time|**10 to 15 minutes**
Nut. Content (per serving): Cal|**511**   Fat|**44.2g**   Protein|**24.5g**   Carbs|**2.54g**

1 teaspoon olive oil
1 teaspoon water
1/16 teaspoon onion powder
2 eggs (whole)

2 slices bacon (fat reduced)
Pepper, adjust to preference
Salt, adjust to preference

1. In a pan set on high heat, cook the bacon till crisp. Let cool and then chop into small pieces. In a bowl, whisk the pepper, salt, onion powder, water, and eggs till fluffy and light.
2. In the pan where you cooked the bacon, add 1 teaspoon olive oil. Heat the oil over medium heat till small bubbles appear. Add the egg mixture; stir till the eggs are cooked. Just before removing the eggs from the stovetop, add the bacon; stir till the ingredients are well mixed.
NOTES: You can add your preferred seasoning and some parsley in the egg mixture for a different flavor.

Caramelized Onion, Chicken Liver, & Madeira

Main Dish: Servings|**4**   Prep. Time| **Fifteen to Twenty min.**   Cook Time|**30 to 35 minutes**
Nut. Content (per serving): Cal|**300**   Fat|**19.4g**   Protein|**26.6g**   Carbs|**3.3g**

1 1/4 pounds chicken liver, halved & patted dry
1 egg (hard-boiled)
1/2 cup wine (Madeira), or Port or Sherry wine
1/2 teaspoon liquid sweeteners

1/4 teaspoon pepper
2 tablespoon parsley, chopped
3 onions, thinly sliced
3 tablespoon olive oil
3/4 teaspoon salt

1. Put 2 tablespoons in a frying pan; heat on medium flame. Add the onions; sauté till golden brown. Add 1/8 teaspoon pepper, 1/2 teaspoon salt, and sugar; stir constantly for 15 minutes till caramelized. Remove the pan from the stove; plate the onions.
2. In the same pan, add 1 tablespoon olive oil; heat on high heat. Add the chicken liver; sauté, seasoning with the rest of the pepper and salt in the process. Cook them for around 2 minutes or till both sides are brown but the inside is still pink. Remove the pan from the heat; plate them on top of the caramelized onion.
3. In the same pan, add the wine. Heat and let come to a boil, continuously stirring it for 1 minute. Turn off the flame. Pour the sauce on top of the plated caramelized onion and liver. Garnish with egg and parsley.

Denver Omelet

Breakfast: Servings|**4**   Prep. Time|**15 minutes**   Cook Time|**25 minutes**
Nut. Content (per serving): Cal|**423**   Fat|**28.3g**   Protein|**34.8g**   Carbs|**5.7g**

1 cup cheese (low fat), shredded
1 cup ham, chopped & cooked
1/2 cup milk (skimmed or low-fat)
1/2 cup onion, finely sliced

1/4 cup bell pepper (green), diced
1/4 teaspoon parsley
8 eggs

1. Preheat your oven to 400F. Whisk the milk and eggs till airy and smooth. Add the cheese, onion, parsley, bell pepper, and ham; stir to mix well. Thinly grease your baking dish using olive oil. Add the egg mixture in the dish. Bake for 25 minutes.

Red Wine Stewed Beef

Main Dish: Servings|8   Prep. Time| **Twenty to Twenty-Five min.**   Cook Time| **3 hours**
Nut. Content (per serving): Cal|**677**   Fat|**30g**   Protein|**95g**   Carbs|**7.5g**

1/2 teaspoon pepper
1 3/4 teaspoons salt
1 bay leaf
1 cup wine (dry red)
1 teaspoon paprika
1 turnip, peeled & cubed
1/4 teaspoon thyme (fresh), doubled if preferred

16 ounces baby carrots
2 cans broth (beef)
2 tablespoons olive oil
3 tablespoon coriander powder
4 pounds chuck roast (boneless), cut into small pieces
8 ounces packet preferred mushrooms, halved

1. Pat the meat dry with paper towels. Toss the meat with paprika, pepper, 1 teaspoon salt, and 3 tablespoons coriander powder till well coated. Let stand for a couple of minutes.
2. In a pot (large), heat a little oil over medium heat. Add the meat; cook for 4 to 5 minutes or till both sides are brown. Add the beef broth, 1/2 teaspoon salt, thyme, bay leaf, and wine. Mix and scrape the brown bits off the pot; let come to boil.
3. Once boiling, reduce the heat to a simmer; cook for 1 hour. Add the turnip, carrots, mushrooms, and veggies. Cover and simmer for 1 to 1 1/2 hours more over low heat or till the meat is tender.
4. Ladle a small amount of stew in a bowl. Add the coriander powder and 1/4 teaspoon salt; stir to dissolve. Add to the stew; simmer for 20 minutes or till the stew is thick. Serve hot.

Greek Pepper Lemon Fish

Main Dish: Servings|2   Prep. Time| **Twenty to Twenty-Five min.**   Cook Time| **5 to Ten (10) minutes**
Nut. Content (per serving): Cal|**536**   Fat|**37g**   Protein|**47g**   Carbs|**2.4g**

1 tablespoon lemon juice
1 teaspoon oregano leaves (dried)
1/2 teaspoon black pepper
1/2 teaspoon lemon zest

1/2 teaspoon salt (sea)
1/4 cup olive oil
2 garlic cloves, crushed
2 pieces (1 pound total) fish fillets

1. In a bowl (large), mix the oregano, salt, pepper, lemon zest, lemon juice, garlic, and olive oil for the marinade. Add the fish; very gently toss till well coated with the marinade. Cover the bowl. Refrigerate for Fifteen to Twenty min. to let the fish soak the marinade.
2. Put the fish on a layer of foil; grill or broil for 5 to Ten (10) minutes per side or till cooked through, turning the fish once to prevent them from breaking.

Calamari Salad

Main Dish: Servings|4   Prep. Time|30 to 40 minutes   Cook Time|40 to 60minutes
Nut. Content (per serving): Cal|351   Fat|21g   Protein|28.1g   Carbs|13.2g

1 1/2 pounds squid, cleaned
1 cup parsley, chopped
1 garlic clove, crushed
1 red onion, chopped
1 tablespoon vinegar (red wine)
1/2 teaspoon salt

1/3 cup olive oil
1/4 teaspoon black pepper
2 celery ribs in 1/4 inch pieces
2 cups cherry tomatoes
2 tablespoons lemon juice

1. Wash the squids clean. Pat them dry using napkins or paper towels. Slice the tentacles in half. Slice the bodies crosswise into 1/3-inch wide rings.
2. Boil a pot of salted water. Once boiling, add the squid; cook for 40 to 60 seconds or till opaque, making sure not to overcook them. Immediately drain and transfer the squid to an ice bath to stop cooking. Once the squid is cool, drain excess water and then pat dry. Transfer to bowl.
3. In a different bowl, mix the onion, garlic, lime juice, pepper, salt, and vinegar; let stand for 5 minutes.
4. Add the parsley, celery, and tomatoes to the squid. Add the vinegar mixture; let stand for 15 minutes before serving. This dish is best after 8 hours.
NOTES: Add more spices or seasoning to the squid mixture if desired.

Sour & Spicy Mushroom Soup

Appetizer: Servings|4-6   Prep. Time|15 minutes   Cook Time| Fifteen to Twenty min.
Nut. Content (per 4 servings): Cal|223   Fat|3.3g   Protein|10g   Carbs|47g

1 tablespoon liquid sweetener
2 1/4 ounces cherry tomatoes, halved
2 cups stock (vegetable)
3 1/4 ounces oyster mushrooms, sliced
3 1/4 ounces straw mushrooms, sliced
3 chilies (bird's eye), pressed

3 leaves kaffir lime, finely sliced
3 shallots, crushed
3 tablespoons galangal, chopped
3 tablespoons lemongrass, diagonally sliced
3 tablespoons lime juice
4 tablespoons miso paste

1. In a saucepan (large), mix the stock, mushrooms, chilies, lemon, kaffir leaves, galangal, and garlic; heat and let come to a boil. Once boiling, reduce the heat to a simmer; cook for 4 minutes. Remove from the heat. Add the sweetener, miso paste, and lime juice. Serve hot.

Leek & Smoked Salmon Scramble 16, 18

Breakfast: Servings|**6**   Prep. Time|**15 minutes**   Cook Time| **Fifteen to Twenty min.**
Nut. Content (per serving): Cal|**479**   Fat|**31g**   Protein|**34g**   Carbs|**15g**

1 cup sour cream (fat-free)
1 tablespoon chives, chopped
1 tablespoon olive oil
1 teaspoon salt
1/2 teaspoon salt
12 eggs

12 smoked salmon slices
2 1/4 cups leeks, sliced
2 tablespoon olive oil
2 teaspoons lemon zest
3/4 cup yogurt (low-fat)

1. In a bowl (small), mix the salt, lemon zest, and sour cream till well combined; set aside. You can make this about 4 days ahead of time; just refrigerate.
2. In a frying pan (large), add 2 tablespoons olive oil; heat on medium-high flame. Once heated, add the leeks; cover the pan and sauté for 10 minutes. Add 1 tablespoon more of olive oil. Add the egg mixture; scramble till the eggs are cooked. Serve with sour cream, chives, and smoked salmon.

CONSOLIDATION PHASE

Spicy, Saucy Chicken

Main Dish: Servings | **2**   Prep. Time **Ten (10) minutes**   Cook Time | **70 minutes**
Nut. Content (per serving): Cal | **679**   Fat | **22.7g**   Protein | **103.4g**   Carbs | **9g**

1 cup white wine (tolerated)
1 shallot, chopped
1 tablespoon capers
1 tablespoon mustard (whole grain)
1 teaspoon paprika

4 chicken legs
8 teaspoons sour cream (fat-free)
A couple drops olive oil
Salt & pepper

1. Grease a nonstick pan. Add the shallot and chicken; cook till starting to brown. Add the wine and season with pepper and salt to preference; cook for 1 hour over low heat. Once the sauce is reduced, add the paprika, capers, mustard, and sour cream; stir to mix well. Serve hot.

Asparagus Bacon Spears

Appetizer: Servings | **20**   Prep. Time | **Twenty to Twenty-Five min.**   Cook Time | **Twenty to 25 min.**
Nut. Content (per serving): Cal | **57**   Fat | **5.1g**   Protein | **2.1g**   Carbs | **1g**

8 to 10 slices bacon (fat reduced)

1 pound asparagus

1. Clean the asparagus very well; trim off the edges. Slice the bacon lengthwise into halves. Wrap each asparagus with the bacon, spiraling the strip around the spear and leaving the asparagus tip exposed.
2. Put them on a sheet pan; bake for Twenty to Twenty-Five min. in a preheated 400F oven. Serve hot.
NOTES: If you want the spears spicier, sprinkle with some pepper.

Coriander Sole

Main Dish: Servings | **1**   Prep. Time | **5 minutes**   Cook Time | **15 minutes**
Nut. Content (per serving): Cal | **237**   Fat | **6.4g**   Protein | **41g**   Carbs | **2.3g**

1/2 lemon (3 tablespoons)
2 coriander sprigs (fresh)
2 sole fillets

3 tablespoons white wine (tolerated)
Salt & pepper

1. Mix the lemon juice, wine, pepper, salt, and coriander. Add the sole; make sure to coat well and marinate for 1 to 2 hours. Once marinated, add the fish and the marinade into a nonstick pan; cook till the sole is brown. Serve garnished with a sprinkle of coriander.

Lemon Pie

Dessert; Servings|**6**   Prep. Time **Ten (10) minutes**   Cook Time|**25 minutes**
Nut. Content (per serving): Cal|**183**   Fat|**8.4g**   Protein|**9.4g**   Carbs|**19.8g**

1 lemon, zest only
1/3 cup Splenda or stevia (granulated
sweetener), adjust to preference,
preferably organic stevia (Dukan Diet)
1/4 cup oat bran

2 tablespoons evaporated milk (fat-free)
2 tablespoons wheat bran
3/4 cup sour cream (fat-free)
5 eggs, divided

1. Preheat your oven to 400F. Grease a pie plate or quiche pan with a couple drops olive oil. In a bowl, mix the milk, 2 eggs, wheat bran, and oat bran till well combined. Pour the mixture into the container; bake for 5 minutes.
2. Once cooked, remove from the oven. Reduce the temperature to 350F. Mix everything else in a deep container. Pour the mixture into the pre-baked crust. Bake for 20 minutes. Once cooked, remove from the oven. let cool completely and serve.

Shrimp Deviled Eggs

Appetizer: Servings|**8**   Prep. Time|**20 minutes**   Cook Time|**2 minutes**
Nut. Content (per serving): Cal|**101**   Fat|**5.3g**   Protein|**11g**   Carbs|**1.5g**

1 tablespoon chives (fresh), chopped
1 tablespoon parsley (fresh), chopped
16 bay shrimp, cooked & peeled, divided

2 tablespoons sour cream (fat-free)
4 eggs
Salt & pepper

1. In boiling water; cook the eggs for Ten (10) minutes. Transfer to a strainer; put under running cold water to stop cooking. Peel and set them aside. Divide the shrimp into 2 portions. Chop 1/2 of the shrimps; leave the other half whole.
2. Slice the eggs lengthwise into halves. Scoop out the yolks into a bowl. Reserve 2 of the yolks; discard the 2 remaining yolks or save for other uses. Crush the reserved egg yolks using a fork in a mixing bowl. Add the shrimp, sour cream, and cream, seasoning with pepper and salt to preference. Stuff the egg whites with the shrimp mixture. Top with the reserved whole shrimps. Serve.

Fast Asparagus Soup

Appetizer: Servings|2   Prep. Time| **Ten (10) minutes**   Cook Time|**20 minutes**
Nut. Content (per serving): Cal|**286**   Fat|**17g**   Protein|**18g**   Carbs|**24.4g**

2/3 cup half-&-half (fat-free), tolerated
3 tablespoons parsley (fresh), finely chopped

4 cups water
4 jars asparagus spears (white)
Salt (sea) & pepper, adjust to preference

1. Put the water in a pot. And heat till boiling. Add the asparagus, along with the juices in the jars; simmer for 20 minutes on low heat. Pour the asparagus and cooking liquid in a blender (large). Add the parsley and half-&-half; season with pepper and salt to preference. Blend till the texture is smooth.

Garlicky Chicken

Main Dish: Servings|**2 to 4**   Prep. Time|**0 minutes**   Cook Time|**10 to 15 minutes per batch**
Nut. Content (per 2 servings): Cal|**487**   Fat|**31g**   Protein|**48g**   Carbs|**1.6g**

1 teaspoon onion powder
1 teaspoon salt
2 teaspoons garlic powder

3 tablespoons olive oil
4 chicken breasts (boneless & skinless)

1. In a resealable bag or bowl; mix the garlic powder, onion powder, and salt till well blended. Add the chicken; toss and mix till well coated.
2. In a skillet (large), add the olive oil; heat on high flame. Once the oil begins to bubble, reduce the flame. Add the chicken; cook for 10 to 15 minutes per side or till tender. Serve with fresh lettuce.

Coriander Sole

Main Dish: Servings|**1**   Prep. Time|**5 minutes**   Cook Time|**15 minutes**
Nut. Content (per serving): Cal|**237**   Fat|**6.4g**   Protein|**41g**   Carbs|**2.3g**

1/2 lemon (3 tablespoons)
2 coriander sprigs (fresh)
2 sole fillets

3 tablespoons white wine (tolerated)
Salt & pepper

1. Mix the lemon juice, wine, pepper, salt, and coriander. Add the sole; make sure to coat well and marinate for 1 to 2 hours. Once marinated, add the fish and the marinade into a nonstick pan; cook till the sole is brown. Serve garnished with a sprinkle of coriander.

Lancashire Hotpot

Main Dish: Servings|4   Prep. Time|**18 minutes**   Cook Time|**90 minutes**
Nut. Content (per serving): Cal|**753**   Fat|**41g**   Protein|**62.4g**   Carbs|**36g**

1 tablespoon cornstarch (tolerated)
2 bay leaves
2 cups stock (lamb)
2 onions (large), peeled and chopped
2 pounds lamb (stewing meat), sliced into large cubes
2 strips bacon, (low sodium reduced fat)

2 teaspoons Worcestershire sauce
2 thyme sprigs
28 ounces butternut squash, peeled and sliced
3 1/2 ounces mushrooms, sliced
4 carrots, peeled & sliced
Green cabbage (steamed), to serve

1. Dry sauté the bacon for 2 to 3 minutes in a nonstick pot. Add your lamb; fry for one (1) or two (2) minutes. Stir in the mushrooms, carrots, and onions. Add your stock; let come to boil. Add the thyme, bay leaves, and Worcestershire sauce; simmer for 45 minutes.
2. Preheat your oven to 375F. Mix 1 tablespoon water with the cornstarch till smooth. Stir the slurry in the pot; simmer till thick. Transfer the mixture to a casserole dish.
3. Arrange the butternut slices on top of the lamb mixture, spooning some of the sauce on top of the squash as you layer them. Bake for Twenty to Twenty-Five min. or till the squash is cooked. Serve with the steamed cabbage.

Heavenly Guacamole

Appetizer/Snack: Servings|3   Prep. Time|**1 hour, 15 minutes**   Cook Time|**0 minutes**
Nut. Content (per serving): Cal|**350**   Fat|**30g**   Protein|**5.2g**   Carbs|**24g**

1 lemon, juice only
1 teaspoon garlic, finely chopped
1 teaspoon salt
1/2 cup onion, chopped

2 tomatoes, chopped
3 avocados, peeled, pitted & mashed
3 tablespoon parsley or cilantro, chopped
Pinch cayenne pepper

1. Mix everything using a blender or a fork. Refrigerate for at least 1 hour to meld all the flavors. Add more lemon juice, garlic, herbs, and spice to suit your preference.

Stewed Turkey

Main Dish: Servings|4   Prep. Time|**5 minutes**   Cook Time|**30 minutes**
Nut. Content (per serving): Cal|**614**   Fat|**25g**   Protein|**80g**   Carbs|**16g**

1 pound mushrooms, sliced into chunks
1 tablespoon tomato puree mixed with 1/4
cup water
2 cloves garlic
2 shallots
2 tablespoons white wine

3 pounds turkey breast, sliced into chunks
4 carrots (large), sliced into chunks
4 tomatoes, sliced into chunks
Basil
Pinch salt & pepper

1. Put the turkey in a casserole dish. Add the carrots, mushrooms, and tomatoes. Drizzle the white wine, tomato puree, garlic, shallots, and pepper and salt to preference. Cover the dish; cook for 30 minutes over medium heat.

Mustard Chicken

Main Dish: Servings|8   Prep. Time **Ten (10) minutes**   Cook Time|**120 minutes**
Nut. Content (per serving): Cal|**269**   Fat|**7g**   Protein|**47.2g**   Carbs|**1.4g**

1 tablespoon tarragon
1 tablespoon thyme
1/2 cup water
1/4 cup wine (dry white), tolerated

2 tablespoons mustard
4 pounds chicken (thighs or drumsticks)
4 tablespoons sour cream (fat-free)
Pinch salt & pepper

1. In a pan (nonstick); cook the chicken for 5 minutes or till brown, flipping them occasionally. Once brown, season with pepper and salt to preference, and add the water, tarragon, thyme, and wine. Cover; cook for sixty (60) minutes using low heat.
2. Transfer the chicken on a dish, arrange them and cover to keep warm. Skim the fat off the cooking juices. Add the mustard; stir to mix. Add the sour cream; stir to mix. When ready to serve, pour your sauce over the poultry.

Fast Stewed Turkey

Main Dish: Servings|**2**   Prep. Time **Ten (10) minutes**   Cook Time|**20 minutes**
Nut. Content (per serving): Cal|**441**   Fat|**12.4g**   Protein|**62g**   Carbs|**20g**

1 onion, finely chopped
1 tablespoon cream (fat-free)
1/2 cup chicken broth (low sodium)
14 ounces turkey meat

7 ounces button mushrooms, cleaned & sliced
Salt (sea) & pepper, adjust to preference

1. Cut the turkey into large chunks. Add the turkey in a wok with a bit of oil; stir-fry till starting to brown. Add the mushrooms and onions. Add your stock; cover and let cook for twenty (20) minutes.
2. Reduce the heat. Add the sour cream and season with pepper and salt to preference. Serve with green salad or leafy veggies.

Cajun Spiced Pork Chops

Main Dish: Servings|**2 to 4**   Prep. Time| **Fifteen to Twenty min.**   Cook Time|**8 to Ten (10) minutes**
Nut. Content (per serving): Cal|**492**   Fat|**17g**   Protein|**79g**   Carbs|**2g**

1 1/2 teaspoon olive oil
1 teaspoon paprika
1/2 teaspoon cumin powder
1/2 teaspoon garlic salt

1/2 teaspoon powdered black pepper
1/2 teaspoon powdered cayenne pepper
1/2 teaspoon sage (dried)
4 pork chops (center-cut)

1. In a bowl (small), mix the sage, paprika, cayenne, black pepper, cumin, and garlic salt as your marinade. Generously coat the pork with the spice mixture; let sit for 10 to 15 minutes or up to overnight in the fridge to let the meat absorb the flavors.
2. Put the olive oil in a pan (large); heat over high heat. Once small bubbles start to appear, reduce the heat to medium. Add the pork; cook for 8 to Ten (10) minutes total or 4 to 5 minutes per side or till the meat is cooked through. The internal temperature should be at least 63C or 145F for medium-rare doneness.

Easy Peasy Rib Roast II

Main Dish: Servings|**10**   Prep. Time|**2 hours, 15 minutes**   Cook Time|**3 hours & 30 minutes**
Nut. Content (per serving): Cal|**764**   Fat|**67.5g**   Protein|**36g**   Carbs|**2.5g**

1 standing (about 5 pounds) rib roast beef
1 teaspoon garlic powder

1 teaspoon powdered black pepper
2 teaspoons salt

1. Let the beef stand for 1 hour at room temperature before using to help cook it evenly. Preheat your oven to 190F or 375F. Take an oven dish (large), put the ribs in with the ribs under.
2. In a bowl (small), mix the garlic, black pepper, and salt till well combined. Liberally season the ribs with the seasoning mix, making sure it is coated evenly. Cook your ribs in your oven for one (1) hour. After one (1) hour, turn your oven off - do not disturb or open your oven. Let the ribs stay for 3 hours in the oven.
3. Around 1/2 hour just before serving, set the oven to 190F; heat the meat till the internal temperature is 145F. Once desired meat temperature is achieved, remove from the oven and let sit for Ten (10) minutes. Carve and plate.

Chicken Cacciatore

Main Dish: Servings|6   Prep. Time| **Fifteen to Twenty min.**   Cook Time|**45 to 55 minutes**
Nut. Content (per serving): Cal|**535**   Fat|**26g**   Protein|**51g**   Carbs|**24.3g**

2 pieces (400 grams each) cherry tomatoes (canned)
1 onion, chopped
2 garlic cloves, finely chopped
2 tablespoon olive oil

4 tablespoon cottage cheese (fat-free)
6 chicken breasts (skinless & boneless)
Black pepper, adjust to preference
Few basil leaves
Salt adjust, to preference

1. Preheat your oven to 375F or 190C. In a pan (medium), add 1 tablespoon olive oil. Add the onion; sauté on medium heat. Add the garlic; sauté till the onion is soft.
2. Add the tomatoes; cook for 10 to 15 minutes on medium heat or till they are softened. Season with pepper and salt to preference. Once the tomatoes are done, transfer the contents to a bowl. Add the cheese and basil; stir to mix and set aside.
3. In the same pan, heat 2 tablespoons olive oil. Add the chicken and fry till both sides are golden brown. Transfer the chicken to a baking dish. Pour the tomato sauce on top of the chicken; bake at 375F for 25 to 30 minutes. Garnish with some basil leaves; serve hot.

Oysters Kilpatrick

Appetizer: Servings|**4**   Prep. Time|**15 minutes**   Cook Time|**5 to 8 minutes**
Nut. Content (per serving): Cal|**386**   Fat|**20g**   Protein|**33g**   Carbs|**19.4g**

175 grams bacon (fat reduced), chopped
2 cups salt (sea)
2 tablespoons Worcestershire sauce

2 tablespoons parsley, chopped
24 oysters, shucked
Lemon wedges

1. Preheat your grill to medium-high heat before starting on this dish. Put the salt in a baking tray (large) to form a thick layer. Arrange the oyster on their shells on top of the salt. Drizzle the oysters with a little Worcestershire sauce. Top each with a little bacon.
2. Put the baking tray on the grill; cook for 5 to 8 minutes or till the bacon is nicely crisp. Once the oysters are cooked, garnish with parsley. Serve with wedges of lemon.

Tarragon Dressed Pear & Chicken Salad

Main Dish: Servings|**4**   Prep. Time| **Twenty to Twenty-Five min.**   Cook Time|**3 to 4 minutes**
Nut. Content (per serving): Cal|**492**   Fat|**27**   Protein|**54g**   Carbs|**7g**

1 bunch watercress, cleaned & leaves picked
1 lettuce, cleaned & torn
1 pear (ripe), peeled, pitted, & thinly sliced
1 tablespoon olive oil
1 tablespoon tarragon (fresh), chopped
1 tablespoon vinegar (white balsamic)
1 teaspoon liquid sweeter
1/2 cup parsley, chopped

2 fillets (around 500 grams each) chicken breast
2 tablespoon lemon juice
2 teaspoons mustard (whole)
50 grams onion sprouts
Black pepper, adjust to preference
Cooking spray (olive oil)
Salt adjust, to preference

1. Season the chicken with pepper and salt. Over medium flame/heat, heat a frying pan, greasing it with a little oil to coat the pan. Add the chicken; cook each side for 3 to 4 minutes, making sure they are cooked through. Once cooked, let rest for 5 minutes before slicing across into thin pieces; set aside.
2. In a bowl (small), whisk the pepper and salt to preference, sweetener, mustard, tarragon, olive oil, balsamic vinegar, and lemon juice as your dressing. In a bowl (large), toss the chicken, parsley, onion sprout, pear, lettuce, and watercress. Drizzle the dressing over the mixture. Serve.

Tomato Brochette

Appetizer: Servings|**12**   Prep. Time| **Fifteen to Twenty min.**   Cook Time|**2 to 4 minutes**
Nut. Content (per serving): Cal|**131**   Fat|**4g**   Protein|**8.3g**   Carbs|**16.6g**

1 cup mozzarella cheese (fat-free), shredded
1 loaf bread (whole-grain)
1 tablespoon balsamic vinegar
1/2 cup tomatoes (sun-dried), chopped
1/4 cup basil leaves

1/4 teaspoon powdered black pepper
1/4 teaspoon salt
2 tablespoon olive oil
3 cloves garlic, finely chopped
6 tomatoes, finely chopped

1. Preheat your oven to the broiler setting. Cut your bread into thick slices; put them in a baking tray. In a bowl (large), mix pepper and salt to preference, basil leaves, balsamic vinegar, olive oil, garlic, sun-dried tomatoes, and tomatoes till well mixed and flavors melded.
2. Broil the bread for 1 to 2 minutes or just till browned. Spoon the tomato mixture into each bread slice. Top with the mozzarella cheese; broil for 1 to 2 minutes or till the cheese is just melted.

Tuscan Pasta

Main Dish: Servings|**6**   Prep. Time| **Fifteen to Twenty min.**   Cook Time|**30 to 35 minutes**
Nut. Content (per serving): Cal|**224**   Fat|**6.4g**   Protein|**7.8g**   Carbs|**38.2g**

1 onion, finely chopped
1 pound zucchini, sliced
1/2 teaspoon powdered black pepper
1/2 teaspoon salt
2 tablespoon olive oil
2 teaspoon garlic powder
2 teaspoon Italian seasoning

28 ounces (canned) chopped tomatoes
6 ounces pasta (whole grain), cooked & drained
8 ounces (canned) tomato sauce (sugar-free)
8 ounces mushrooms, sliced

1. Set a skillet over medium heat; add the tomatoes, garlic powder, tomato sauce, salt, black pepper, and Italian seasoning; let come to a boil. Once boiling, reduce the heat to low. Cover the pan; simmer for 20 minutes.
2. In a different pan, add the onion; sauté for a couple of minutes. Add the mushroom and zucchini; cook for 4 minutes or till they are crisped. Once they are cooked, add them to the tomato mixture; stir to mix and coat the veggies. Add the pasta; stir to mix. Serve. Sprinkle with shredded cheese if desired.

STABILIZATION PHASE

Pumpkin Bread (Whole-Wheat)

Breakfast: Servings|**12**   Prep. Time|**2 1/2 to 3 hours**   Cook Time|**40 minutes**
Nut. Content (per serving): Cal|**208**   Fat|**9.2g**   Protein|**9.7g**   Carbs|**25g**

1 1/2 cups pumpkin (canned)
1 egg
1 packet active dry yeast
1 tablespoon pumpkin pie spice
1 teaspoon salt

1 teaspoon sugar
1/2 cup evaporated milk (low fat), warmed
3 cup flour (whole wheat)
Cooking spray

1. In a bowl (large), mix the sugar, yeast, and milk till well blended. Let rest for Ten (10) minutes and the yeast starts to act, creating froth. Once the mixture is foamy, add the pumpkin and egg; whisk till well mixed.
2. In a different bowl (large), mix the salt and flour. Add the wet ingredients into the dry ingredients; mix and knead till it forms a smooth dough. Dust a clean cooking board or counter pot with some dry flour; knead the dough for 2 to 3 minutes.
3. Line a bowl with a little cooking spray; transfer the dough in the bowl. Turn the dough to coat all the sides with the cooking spray evenly. Cover the dough with a damp kitchen towel. Place in a warm area for 1 to 1 1/2 hours till the size doubles. Once the sized doubles, remove the towel; punch down the dough with your fist before removing from the bowl.
4. Shape the dough into a rough cylinder form, making sure it will fit in your loaf pan. With the seam side above, put the dough in the pan, ensuring the sides of the dough touches the tin. Cover with a damp kitchen towel; let sit for 30 to 60 minutes or till the size doubles.
5. Preheat your oven to 190C or 375F. Bake the dough for 40 minutes or till golden brown. The bread is done when it sounds hollow when you tap the crust. Transfer the loaf pan to a cooling rack. Once the bread is cooled, remove the bread to a cooling rack; let completely cool before slicing.
NOTES: Do not eat more than 2 slices a day.

Shrimp Cocktail

Main Dish: Servings|**2 to 4**   Prep. Time **Ten (10) minutes**   Cook Time|**0 minutes**
Nut. Content (per 2 servings): Cal|**330**   Fat|**1.5g**   Protein|**48g**   Carbs|**31.3g**

1 pound shrimp, shelled, deveined, & cooked
1 teaspoon Worcestershire sauce (sugar-free or low sugar)

1/2 cup chili sauce
1/2 cup diet ketchup
3 teaspoons horseradish

1. In a small bowl, mix the horseradish, ketchup, and chili sauce in a bowl (small) till well blended. Serve with the shrimp.

Stir-Fried Chinese Chicken

Main Dish: Servings|**4**   Prep. Time| **Twenty to Twenty-Five min.**   Cook Time| **Fifteen to Twenty min.**
Nut. Content (per serving): Cal|**512**   Fat|**26g**   Protein|**48.4g**   Carbs|**22.2g**

1 1/2 cups chicken broth (hot)
1 bell pepper (red), thinly sliced
1 broccoli, divided into small florets
1 cup Chinese cabbage or bok choy, sliced
1 onion, diced
1 tablespoon ginger, finely chopped
1/2 cauliflower, separated small florets
1/2 cup mushrooms, finely sliced
1/2 pound asparagus
1/2 pound green beans

2 bell peppers (green), thinly sliced
2 carrots, sliced into matchsticks
2 celery stalks, sliced
2 cloves garlic, finely chopped
2 tablespoons cornstarch
2 tablespoons hot water
2 tablespoons olive oil
2 tablespoons soy sauce
3 spring onions, sliced
4 chicken breasts (boneless & skinless)

1. In a bowl (large), put the bok choy, asparagus, green beans, cauliflower, and broccoli. Add the boiling water; let rest for 2 minutes. Drain and set aside till use. Slice the chicken into small chunks.
2. Over a medium flame, heat a wok. Add 2 tablespoons olive oil and the chicken; fry for 4 minutes or till golden brown or cooked. Add the red and green peppers and carrots; sauté for a couple of minutes. Add the mixed veggies; drizzle the soy sauce over them. Stir-fry for 4 minutes or till the veggies are cooked.
3. Mix the cornstarch with 2 tablespoons hot water till smooth. Add the slurry in the wok. Add the broth. Cover the wok; cook for 3 minutes. Serve with cooked rice (whole-grain) or alone.

White Wine Mushroom

Appetizer: Servings|**3**   Prep. Time|**10 to 15 minutes**   Cook Time| **Fifteen to Twenty min.**
Nut. Content (per serving): Cal|**111**   Fat|**5.6g**   Protein|**5.3g**   Carbs|**14g**

2 tablespoons chives, chopped
2 cloves garlic, finely chopped
1/4 cup wine (dry white)

1 teaspoon Italian seasoning
1 tablespoon olive oil
1 1/2 pounds white mushrooms

1. Put 1 tablespoon olive oil in a skillet; set the flame to medium heat. Add the mushrooms and Italian seasoning; sauté for Ten (10) minutes, constantly stirring to prevent them from sticking to the bottom of the skillet.
2. Add the garlic and wine; cook for 1 to 2 minutes till the wine is completely evaporated and the mushrooms are cooked. Adjust pepper and salt to preference as needed. Garnish with the chives; stir to mix and serve.

Crusted Tofu &Vegetables

Main Dish: Servings|4   Prep. Time|**20 minutes**   Cook Time|**25 to 30 minutes**
Nut. Content (per serving): Cal|**449**   Fat|**33.4g**   Protein|**22g**   Carbs|**22g**

Other ingredients:
1 bunch Chinese cabbage or bok choy
1 Jalapeno pepper, sliced
1 sweet red bell pepper, sliced
1 tablespoon cornstarch
1 tablespoon soy sauce
1/2 tablespoon miso paste
1/2 tablespoon wine vinegar
1-inch ginger, finely chopped
2 carrots, sliced into matchsticks
2 cloves garlic, finely chopped
2 tablespoons olive oil

2 to 3 spring onions, finely sliced
3 tablespoons water

Tofu & marinade:
4 garlic cloves, finely chopped
1/2 tablespoon wine vinegar
1/2 tablespoon olive oil
1 tablespoon soy sauce
1 tablespoon miso paste
1 packet tofu, drained & patted dried
1-inch ginger, finely chopped

1. Slice the tofu into 1-inch cubes. In a bowl (medium), mix the ginger, garlic, olive oil, miso paste, vinegar, and soy sauce as your marinade. Add the tofu in the bowl; toss and stir till they are coated evenly. Refrigerate to marinate for 15 minutes up to overnight.
2. In a saucepan (large), heat 1 tablespoon olive oil on medium heat. When bubbles start to appear, add the tofu and marinade; cook for 8 to ten (10) minutes or till all the sides are golden brown. Transfer your tofu to a paper towel-covered plate to absorb excess oil.
3. Using the pan again; warm 1 tablespoon of olive oil. Once the oil is hot enough, add the ginger, spring onion, jalapeno, and garlic; sauté for 2 minutes or till done. Add the carrots, peppers, and celery; sauté for 3 to 5 minute or till the veggies are crisped tender. Add the bok choy; cook for 3 to 5 minutes or till they are wilted.
4. Mix the water, cornstarch, olive oil, vinegar, miso paste, and soy sauce till blended. Add the mixture to the pan; cook for 2 minutes or till the sauce is thick. Add the tofu. Serve.
NOTES: Add more soy sauce if you cannot find miso paste.

Tomato and Bresaola Salad

Appetizer: Servings|4   Prep. Time|**15 minutes**   Cook Time|**0 minutes**
Nut. Content (per serving): Cal|**500**   Fat|**25g**   Protein|**60g**   Carbs|**12g**

1 tablespoon olive oil
40 bresaola slices
8 to 10 leaves basil

8 to 9 ounces cheese (Bulgarian feta, low fat)
8 tomatoes, finely sliced into thin circles

1. In a tray (flat), arrange the tomato slices side by side to create a layer. Layer the bresaola on top of the tomato layer. Distribute the cheese on top. Drizzle with a little olive oil. Serve.

Easy Planked Cedar Salmon

Main Dish: Servings|6   Prep. Time|25 to 30 minutes   Cook Time|20minutes
Nut. Content (per serving): Cal|614   Fat|36.4g   Protein|64g   Carbs|4g

1 1/2 teaspoons vinegar (rice wine)
1 tablespoon ginger paste
1 teaspoon garlic paste
1 teaspoon sesame seed oil
1/3 cup olive oil

1/3 cup soy sauce
1/4 cup green onions, chopped
2 piece (2 pounds each) salmon fillets
3 pieces (12-inch long) cedar planks, untreated

1. Before cooking, soak the cedar months with warm water for 1 hour or longer if possible. Mix the garlic paste, ginger, green onion, soy sauce, both oils, and vinegar till well blended as your marinade. Add the fish, coat well with the marinade, and let rest for 15 minutes.
2. Meanwhile, preheat your grill to medium heat. Put the planks on the grill. They are ready once they start to smoke. Put the fish on the planks. Cover the grill and cook for 20 minutes or till the fish is cooked.

Tasty Thai Chicken Soup

Main Dish: Servings|2 to 4   Prep. Time| Fifteen to Twenty min.   Cook Time|20 to 30 minutes
Nut. Content (per 4 servings): Cal|172   Fat|7.1g   Protein|20g   Carbs|9.7g

1 chicken breast, halved & shredded
1 coriander sprig (fresh), chopped
1 tablespoon fish sauce
1 tablespoon lime juice
1 tablespoon tom yum paste
1 teaspoon chili pepper (green), chopped

1/2 clove garlic, chopped
2 leaves Kaffir lime
3 cups stock (chicken)
3 stalks lemongrass, sliced
4 ounces mushrooms, sliced
4 to 5 leaves basil (fresh), chopped

1. Put the stock in a pot (large); heat and let come to a boil. Add the tom yum and garlic; cook for 1 to 2 minutes. Add the lime leaves and lemongrass. Once fragrant, add the lemongrass and chicken; cook till the chicken is tender.
2. Add the mushrooms, chili pepper, and fish sauce. Add the lime juice and coriander. Serve hot.

Bacon-y Brussels Sprouts

Appetizer: Servings|6   Prep. Time| **Fifteen to Twenty min.**   Cook Time| **25 to 30 minutes**
Nut. Content (per serving): Cal| **223**   Fat| **14.4g**   Protein| **9.9g**   Carbs| **18g**

1 1/2 pounds Brussels sprouts, trimmed & halved
1 tablespoon olive oil
1/2 cup balsamic vinegar

1/2 pounds bacon, chopped
1/4 onion, finely chopped
2 cups chicken stock
2 garlic cloves, minced

1. In a skillet (large), cook the bacon for Ten (10) minutes or till brown and crisp. Transfer your bacon to your paper towel-covered plate. Remove the bacon grease from the skillet.
2. Add 1 tablespoon olive oil in the skillet. Add the garlic and onion; sauté for 5 to 7 minutes or till softened. Season with pepper and salt to preference. Add 1/2 cup balsamic vinegar; let come to a boil. Simmer till 1/3 of the vinegar has evaporated.
3. Add your stock, bacon, and Brussels sprouts; increase the flame to high and let come to a boil. Once boiling, reduce the flame to medium; simmer for Ten (10) minutes or till the Brussels sprouts are cooked.

Tasty Basil Thai Chicken

Main Dish: Servings|6   Prep. Time| **40 to 45 minutes**   Cook Time| **1 hour**
Nut. Content (per serving): Cal| **298**   Fat| **11g**   Protein| **45g**   Carbs| **3.1g**

1 lemon, zest, and juice
1 teaspoon ginger paste
2 tablespoons fish sauce
2 tablespoons soy sauce
2 tablespoons yogurt (low fat)

2 teaspoons flakes red pepper
3 cloves garlic, finely minced
3 pounds chicken thighs, skinless
3 tablespoons basil, finely minced

1. In a resealable bag, mix the ginger paste, red pepper, basil, garlic, lemon zest, lemon juice, yogurt, fish sauce, and soy sauce till well blended. Add the chicken, seal, and toss and shake the bag to coat well. Let marinate at room temperature for 30 minutes or marinate overnight in the fridge.
2. Preheat to 190C or 375F. Transfer the chicken and marinade in a baking dish. Bake for 1 hour or till the chicken is cooked and juicy.

Conclusion

Valuable information and details about the Dukan Diet for newbies will help you start on the eating habit and begin creating a suitable menu. A simple run-down of the four phases and important pointers of the plan will help you understand the basics so that you can successfully adopt the changes.

It also helps that recipes are categorized by phase – Attack, Cruise, Consolidation, and Stabilization - and indicated for which part of the meal plan you can serve them. Reading about the various tips will help you easily prepare, maximize the recipes, and even adopt classic dishes for your diet. You will also have a 21-day head start with the well-laid menu.

Interested in becoming a master chef? ;)

If you liked the recipes in this book, then you might be interested in the following books.

Dash Slow Cooker Cookbook
Link to Amazon:
https://amzn.to/2XK6XYW

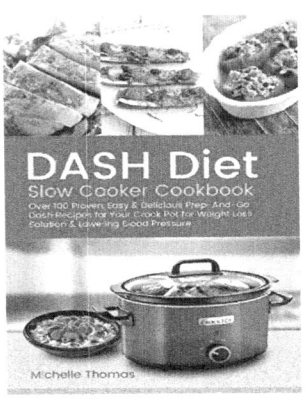

Anti-Inflammatory Diet Instant Pot
Cookbook Link to Amazon:
https://amzn.to/2TrBkoL

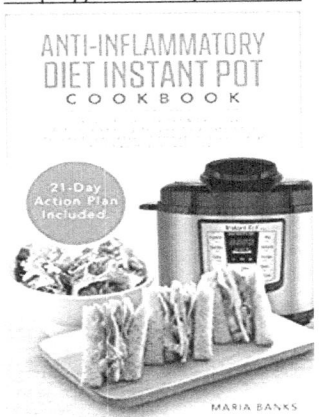

Prediabetes Cookbook
Link to Amazon:
https://amzn.to/2XMtC7i

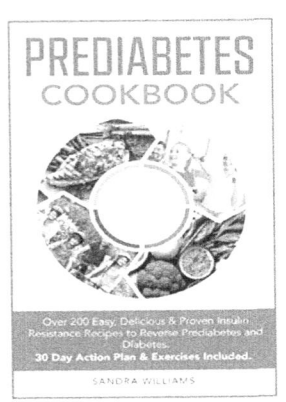

Mind Diet Cookbook
Link to Amazon:
https://amzn.to/2Ttctke

Dash Cookbook
Link to Amazon:
https://amzn.to/2HgXGly

Keto Fat Bombs Cookbook
Link to Amazon:
https://amzn.to/2Cb7t9A

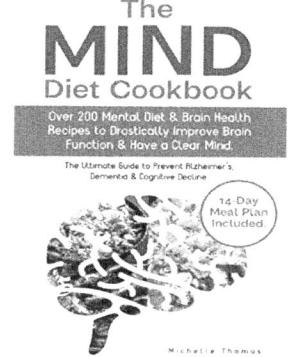

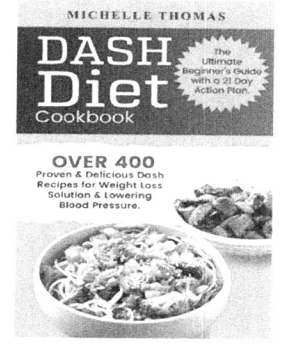

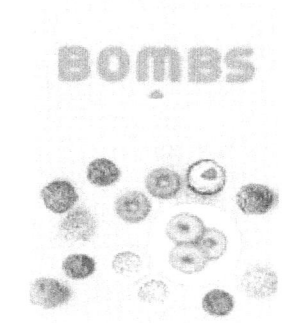

Type 2 Diabetes Cookbook
Link to Amazon:
https://amzn.to/2Uqzzo8

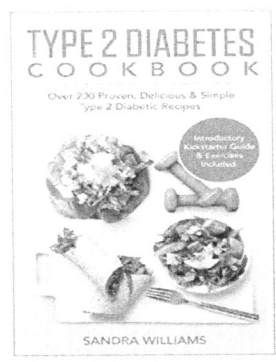

PCOS Cookbook
Link to Amazon:
https://amzn.to/2tYbOsc

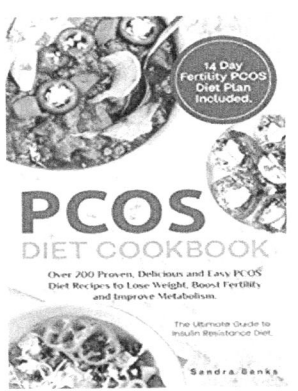

Lectin Free Diet Cookbook
Link to Amazon:
https://amzn.to/2XMqxUl

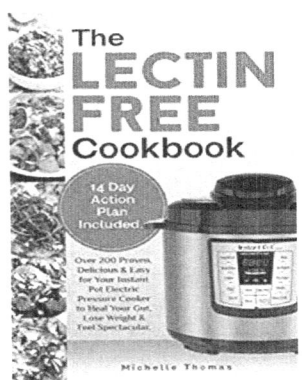

Dukan Diet Cookbook
Link to Amazon:
https://amzn.to/2EPmXjO

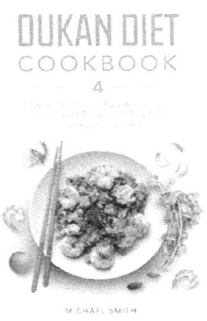

Mini Instant Pot Cookbook
Link to Amazon:
https://amzn.to/2NQXo68

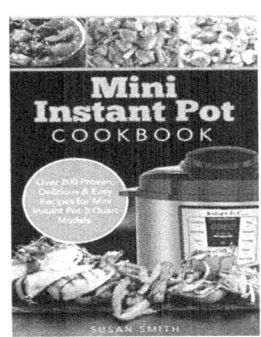

We sincerely hope you enjoyed the recipes.

If you feel like we could improve the cookbook please email us at info@limitlessrecipes.com and we'll make sure to get back to you.

We have a big passion for cooking and we love writing cookbooks but quite often it's pretty hard to compete with all the big publishing companies out there. Reviews really help us and we would appreciate it if you could take a minute and leave a review of the book.

If you could take one minute to leave a review, we would really appreciate that.

You can also leave a review by following these 3 steps:

1. Go to the product page

2. Scroll down and on the left side click 'Write customer review'

3. Write a review and click 'Submit'

Thank you, it really means a lot. Who's amazing? You are!

Final Words

Thank you again for downloading this book!

I hope this book was able to help you start a wonderful adventure in the kitchen making delicious and healthy home-cooked Dukan Diet meals. I also hope you enjoyed reading and trying out all the wonderful dishes.

I also hope you learned a great value about the 4 phases of this eating habit, the 100 approved foods on the diet, and loved the recipes. Happy Dukan Diet cooking!

60274687R00046